THE ENDURING SELF IN PEOPLE WITH ALZHEIMER'S

THE ENDURING SELF IN PEOPLE WITH ALZHEIMER'S

GETTING TO THE HEART OF INDIVIDUALIZED CARE

BY
SAM FAZIO, PH.D.

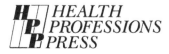

HEALTH
PROFESSIONS
PRESS

BALTIMORE • LONDON • SYDNEY

169452515   4-16-09

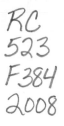

**HEALTH
PROFESSIONS
PRESS**

Health Professions Press, Inc.
Post Office Box 10624
Baltimore, Maryland 21285-0624

www.healthpropress.com

Typeset by Karen Wenk.
Manufactured in the United States of America by Maple-Vail, York, PA.
Cover and interior designs by Tony Olivis.

The information provided in this book is in no way meant to substitute for a medical practitioner's advice or expert opinion. Readers should consult a medical practitioner if they are interested in more information on Alzheimer's disease. This book is sold without warranties of any kind, express or implied, and the publisher and author disclaim any liability, loss, or damage caused by the contents of this book.

Library of Congress Cataloging-in-Publication Data

Fazio, Sam.
   The enduring self in people with Alzheimer's : getting to the heart of individualized care / by Sam Fazio.
      p. ; cm.
   Includes bibliographical references and index.
   ISBN-13: 978-1-932529-38-8 (pbk.)
   1. Alzheimer's disease—Patients—Care. 2. Caregivers—Psychology. 3. Self-perception. I. Title.
   [DNLM: 1. Alzheimer Disease—nursing. 2. Alzheimer Disease—psychology. 3. Caregivers—psychology. 4. Self Concept. WT 155 F287e 2008]
   RC523.F384 2008
   362.196'831—dc22
                                    2007035750

British Library of Cataloguing-in-Publication data are available from the British Library.

CONTENTS

About the Author vii

Foreword by
Stephen Post ix

Preface xi

Acknowledgments xiii

Introduction 1

Section I: A Framework for Understanding the Self in Alzheimer's Care

CHAPTER ONE: The Self as the Core of Person-Centered Care 5

CHAPTER TWO: Overview of Self 33

CHAPTER THREE: Overview of Alzheimer's Disease 43

CHAPTER FOUR: Evidence of the Self in Alzheimer's Disease 57

Section II: Essential Elements of Care that Support Selfhood

CHAPTER FIVE: Physical and Social Environments that
Recognize the Self 75

CHAPTER SIX: Relationships and Interactions that
Support the Self 99

Section III: Key Concepts for Maintaining the Self

CHAPTER SEVEN: Supporting the Self in Everyday Care 115

CHAPTER EIGHT: Sharing the Self with Others 133

Appendix: Research Method and Results 149

References 157

Recommended Readings 165

Index 169

ABOUT THE AUTHOR

Sam Fazio has a doctorate in developmental psychology from Loyola University Chicago. He has worked for the national headquarters of the Alzheimer's Association since 1994 in a variety of areas, including Education and Training and Program Services. He currently works in the Medical and Scientific Relations area, overseeing the international research conferences, scientific journal, and social/behavioral research initiatives. Dr. Fazio also is involved in several research projects with older adults in the Chicago area related to the persistence of self, person-centered care, and health and wellness.

Prior to working for the Alzheimer's Association, Dr. Fazio worked for Rush Presbyterian–St. Luke's Medical Center at the Alzheimer's Family Care Center, an adult day center specifically designed for people with dementia. He has been in the field of aging since 1987 and has a broad range of experience that includes leadership and management roles, working with older adults and families, and providing direct care. He has presented both nationally and internationally and has published several journal articles and book chapters. Dr. Fazio is also the co-author of the book *Rethinking Alzheimer's Care* (1999, Health Professions Press).

FOREWORD

Across North America and Europe a movement is afoot to revolutionize the ways in which we think about and care for the deeply forgetful. For many decades, older adults have rightly extracted a promise from their loved ones: "Please, never put me in a nursing home!" This is because the nursing home model did little more than warehouse older adults, especially those who had any degree of memory deficit, and treated them entirely in terms of a medical care model that focused only on their physical needs. Overly objective and pacifying, this model tends to treat older adults as biological substrates rather than as human beings capable of choice, purpose, creativity, prosocial activities, and meaningful emotion and relationality. No wonder older adults have feared the "nursing home" fate. Fortunately there has been a major grass roots effort to change from a *medical* to a *person-centered* model of care that takes older adults—including the deeply forgetful—seriously as active agents in daily life. Organizations such as the Pioneer Network have fostered a culture change that enhances the lives of older adults within environments that respect and nurture their remaining capacities. In other words, the older adult with dementia is a glass half full rather than half empty, and is worthy of being treated as a person rather than a mere biological object.

There have been several notable leaders in this movement, and certainly Sam Fazio is one of them. For the past decade, Sam has been right at the center of this powerful movement to create institutions and forms of care that treat the person as a person. In this wonderful book, *The Enduring Self in People with Alzheimer's*, he has synthesized a wealth of knowledge about the very nature of the enduring self with dementia, and he has coupled this with a hands-on knowledge of all the best approaches to forms of care that enable this self to flourish emotionally, relationally, and physically. With the publication of this book, Sam Fazio stands alongside luminaries in the field including Tom Kitwood, Rose Marie Fagan, Steven Sabat, and Steve Shields, all of whom have contributed powerfully to a new vision of living with deep forgetfulness in ways that validate and redeem.

Despite the seriousness of dementia and the responsibilities it creates for caregivers, it is ethically important not to judge the person with dementia by "hypercognitive" values. A bias against deeply forgetful individuals is inevitable in theories of moral status in which persons are defined only by the presence of a set of cognitive abilities. Rationality is too severe a ground for moral standing, allowing if not requiring the relational and emotional deaths of many individuals who may, in fact, continue to enjoy simple pleasures despite their lack of rationality. The self is not cognition alone, but is rather a complex entity with emotional and relational aspects that should be deemed morally significant and worthy of affirmation.

The fitting moral response to people with dementia within classical western ethical thought and related conceptions of common human decency, then, is to enlarge our sense of human worth in a way that will counter the exclusionary emphasis on traits such as rationality, efficient use of time and energy, ability to control distracting impulses, thrift, economic success, self-reliance, self-control, "language advantage," and the like. The perils of forgetfulness are especially evident in our culture of independence and economic productivity, which so values intellect, memory, and self-control. Looking beyond these cognitive traits, it is possible for emotional, relational, aesthetic, and symbolic well-being to be experienced and expressed to varying degrees in people with progressive dementia. The first crucial step in enhancing quality of life is accepting the reality of the person with dementia rather than trying to impose one's own reality. In general, quality of life is a self-fulfilling prophesy. If those around the person with dementia see the glass as half empty and make no effort to relate to the person in ways that enhance his or her experience, then quality of life is minimal.

Sam Fazio provides us with the finest moral, psychological, and practical book yet available on how to recognize, acknowledge, and support in countless practical ways the enduring self underlying the losses that Alzheimer's disease inevitably brings. In so doing, he makes a significant contribution to improving the quality of life of people with dementia. This elegantly written and remarkably clear book will serve as the gold standard for those who wish to maintain the dignity and humanity of the deeply forgetful.

Stephen G. Post, Ph.D.
Professor, School of Medicine
Case Western Reserve University

PREFACE

In 1987, I was first introduced to Alzheimer's disease when my internship supervisor was being transferred from a skilled nursing facility to a new adult day center, the Alzheimer's Family Care Center, that was being developed for people with Alzheimer's disease. I eagerly went along, not knowing a thing about Alzheimer's disease. I quickly read everything I could about the disease (which was not much) so that I could be as informed as possible going into my new role. The small amount of information I was able to find seemed different from what I was seeing and experiencing firsthand at the day center. The best and most accurate learning, however, took place from being with the people with the disease and from seeing how the staff interacted with, cared for, and supported each of them in their own way. People were relating in genuine, caring, and authentic ways—ways I had not seen before in care environments. It was so comfortable to be there and, in a sense, it was even magical. I felt a connection with these individuals that I had never felt before. It was then that I knew this was the right place for me.

My experiences at the Alzheimer's Family Care Center have had a significant impact on my growth and development. It was there that I was supported and challenged to be a better carer and to find ways to truly meet the needs, interests, and strengths of each individual. It was there that I developed an overall philosophical approach to dementia care and an expertise that could be shared with others in a variety of ways. It was there that I learned to truly appreciate people with dementia.

This book is a culmination of the last 20 years. It includes content I have gleaned from individuals and families I have known, from what I learned at the day center and at the Alzheimer's Association, from ideas discussed by experts and colleagues, and from various bodies of literature. It attempts to summarize current research, practice, and thinking related to the self and to Alzheimer's care. It also includes and expands on thoughts that were introduced in my earlier coauthored book *Rethinking Alzheimer's Care*, thoughts that are essential to good person-centered care. At the same time, it includes new research I conducted on the persistence of self and translates that research into practice.

This book represents a continuation of my interest in and passion for care that is reflective of the whole person. I use research as the foundation to develop discussions and practical applications in everyday care and interactions. This book does not necessarily provide answers, but rather continues to explore and clarify the themes of good dementia care. I hope this book will encourage you to rethink your programs, care, and interactions to ensure that the whole person is always recognized and supported.

ACKNOWLEDGMENTS

I would like to begin by acknowledging all of the individuals with dementia who I have had the privilege to know over the past 20 years. These individuals have taught me more about life and care than any school or book ever could. They have inspired me to develop a vocation rather than a profession, and to expand my overall approach and philosophy to the world. The same is true for the families I have known and worked with over the years. I truly appreciate their openness, honesty, and willingness to spend time with me and to allow me to learn from them.

There have been many friends, colleagues, and mentors who have been supportive over the years and who have been *comrades of consciousness* throughout this 20-year journey, most specifically Dorothy Seman and Jane Stansell, my co-authors for *Rethinking Alzheimer's Care*. There are even others who have not known that they have been instrumental in my thoughts and work, but who have been from afar, especially Steven Sabat and Tom Kitwood. In addition, there are many other colleagues committed to dementia research and care who I have met over the years and who have influenced me in many ways. Unfortunately, I do not have enough room to recognize each of them.

The Alzheimer's Association has also been a great support in my professional development. I especially appreciate the opportunities I have had within the organization and the flexibility that its leaders have allowed me so that I can continue to grow professionally. Loyola University Chicago also has been a great support in my professional growth. I would especially like to recognize Dr. David Mitchell and Dr. Catherine Haden for their interest in my work and for their involvement and mentorship. At the same time, I would like to thank the individuals, families, and organizations who were a part of my research.

I would also like to thank my family and friends for their ongoing support, encouragement, and overall tolerance. Finally and importantly, I would like to acknowledge each of you for the work you do every day to make your community and the world a better place for people with Alzheimer's disease—a place that recognizes and supports the whole self of each individual.

INTRODUCTION

Over the past decade there has been an abundance of information about good dementia care produced by a variety of people and housed in a variety of places. Much of that information shares common elements regarding how to provide care that supports the person. I decided to write this book to revisit that information, specifically in relation to the preservation of self, and to put much of that good information in one place. My current research regarding the persistence of self also adds a new dimension to this ongoing discussion. This book was designed to highlight various theoretical and philosophical perspectives, review research and evidence, and illustrate how they can all be translated into practice and applied to our everyday care approaches and interactions.

The book is divided into three major sections. Section I provides the foundation with background on the self, Alzheimer's disease, and person-centered care. Chapter One reviews the fundamental elements of dementia care that support personhood, or the self. Topics include the culture change movement, the impact of language, the concept of caring, core values in providing care, and getting to know the individual with dementia. Chapter Two takes a step back and highlights theories about the self and how it develops with time and experience. Definitions of self, measurements of self, and the evolution and adaptation of self throughout the life course are discussed. Chapter Three then reviews the basics of Alzheimer's disease and evolving thinking about it. Topics include diagnosis and progression, treatment, and models of care. Chapter Four summarizes my research on the persistence of self. The chapter outlines how the self can be measured through language use and visual self-recognition. The data and more specific details about the study are provided in the appendix. Together, the first four chapters provide the background or evidence for practices that support the self in everyday care.

Section II provides a description of essential elements of care that support selfhood. Chapter Five reviews how the physical and interpersonal environments can be structured to support the self. Topics include key principles of design, identity and home, therapeutic milieu, and approaches to activities that recognize the self. Chapter Six then discusses more specifically how interactions and relationships can be approached to honor and maintain the self. The role of the care provider in caring, in listening and communicating, and in deeper caring connections is discussed. Together, these two chapters provide ideas for how thinking and practice can evolve to meet individual needs and to support the self.

Section III brings together the foundation and essential elements that are discussed in the first two sections and outlines the key concepts for maintaining the self. Chapter Seven describes specific elements of care and ways of thinking that sustain the self. Topics in this chapter include maintaining the self, creating supportive environments, being in the moment, and interventions that support identity. Chapter Eight provides action steps and resources to use in sharing the essentials of maintaining selfhood with others in your community. This chapter includes a plan of action and key points from the previous chapters to share with others. Together, these two chapters provide the framework and tools to take the information back to your community and to start, or to continue, the culture change movement.

This book has been designed to include many practical pieces for the reader. Throughout chapters, examples are provided to illustrate concepts. Additionally, each chapter ends with an exercise, or SELF-Reflection, to encourage you to think through the information and to consider how to apply it in your community. A case example is also provided at the end of Chapter Seven to tie all of the concepts together into a real-world example and to bring the entire book to life. Finally, recommended readings are included at the end of the book to share a range of resources that have influenced my thinking and practice.

The purpose of this book is to expand and inspire the continuing discussion of changes in thinking, attitudes, and care approaches in communities that provide care to people with dementia. It hopefully will be a stepping-stone to increasingly better care practices that recognize and support the self. Remember, change takes time and attention. It sometimes requires us to be patient and persistent at the same time. Keep in mind that one small change can have rippling effects and can serve as an example or catalyst for others to follow.

SECTION I

A FRAMEWORK FOR UNDERSTANDING THE SELF IN ALZHEIMER'S CARE

CHAPTER ONE

THE SELF AS THE CORE OF PERSON-CENTERED CARE

Person-Centered Care is high-quality interpersonal care that affirms personhood, resulting in the preservation of self.

Kitwood and Bredin (1992)

Personhood is often seen as synonymous with selfhood, and a fundamental component of person-centered care is honoring the self or the person. In person-centered care, care providers adapt schedules, decision-making processes, approaches to care, and environments to meet the needs, abilities, personality, preferences, and functioning of each individual. This chapter reviews the fundamental aspects of person-centered care and discusses how they are essential in maintaining the self.

Personhood and the Impetus of Person-Centered Care

You cannot discuss the concept of personhood or person-centered care without talking about the work and beliefs of Tom Kitwood, a British psychiatrist known for groundbreaking work assessing the well-being of people with dementia. He proposed that dementia could be best understood as an interplay between neurological impairment (or brain disease) and psychosocial factors, namely health, individual psychology, and the environment, with particular emphasis on social context (Kitwood, 1998). He found that the environment has as much effect on the brain as the brain has on a person's abilities. Neuroscientist Marian Diamond stated a similar belief, that people with a brain disease will be negatively affected at a neurological level by an impoverished environment and will be enhanced by an enriched environment (Downs et al., 2006).

Fundamental to Kitwood's theory was a rejection of the standard medical approach to dementia, which he found to be faulty and deficient. He maintained that the basic assumption in the medical sciences that dementia is caused by diseased neurological processes in a linear fashion was an inadequate explanation for all of the symptoms (expressions) of the disease, and that it carried far too negative and predictable implications for the nature of caregiving (Kitwood & Bredin, 1992).

Kitwood and Bredin (1992) shared evidence from studies of different care practices suggesting that dementia is not necessarily a process of inevitable and general deterioration. It varies from person to person. The person with dementia is in a state of relative well-being or ill-being. Hours of detailed observation evolved into 12 indicators of well-being, which include:

1. Assertion of desire or will

2. Ability to experience and express a range of emotions

3. Initiation of social contact

4. Affectional warmth

5. Social sensitivity

6. Self-respect

7. Acceptance of others with dementia

8. Humor

9. Creativity and self-expression

10. Showing evident pleasure

11. Helpfulness

12. Relaxation

Based on these observations, Kitwood and Bredin suggested that there are four global states of which the indicators are, to varying degrees, an expression. The first global state is a sense of personal worth, which is the deepest level of self-esteem. The second state is a sense of agency, or the ability to control personal life in a meaningful way—to produce, to achieve, to make some mark upon others and the world. The third state is one of social confidence, a feeling of being at ease with others, of being able to move towards them, of having something to offer them. The fourth state is that of hope (Kitwood & Bredin, 1992).

At the core of Kitwood's theories is the belief that human beings are far more deeply affected by the social psychology that surrounds them than is commonly recognized. He discusses the concept of *malignant social psychology*, which will be discussed in Chapter Seven. Each aspect of malignant social psychology is damaging to self-esteem and tends to diminish person-hood. When a person has been subjected to a predominately malignant social psychology for several years, the effects may be devastating. Kitwood and Bredin (1992) stated that the most disabling effects of brain disease are to be found not in functional impairment, but in the threats to one's self and personhood. They maintained that personhood is dependent on other people.

Kitwood and Bredin (1992) developed an assessment and observational tool called *dementia care mapping*, which involves observing several residents in short intervals and coding the observations in relation to the residents' degree of well- or ill-being. The information creates an overall picture of how each person spends his or her day and how he or she feels about it. Kitwood and Bredin observed that residents typically spent long periods of time without any human contact. Even when staff ratios were favorable, it was still common to find that interactions were brief and superficial. Kitwood and Bredin offer three reasons for this: Staff members are rarely trained in how to engage a resident, are typically not fully supported by administrators, and underestimate what people with dementia can do.

A key element of Kitwood's work is the preservation of self. The most central outcome of Kitwood's model is the need for high-quality interpersonal care that affirms personhood, and the approach that he and Bredin developed to fill this need is called *person-centered care*. They looked at what people with dementia need and determined that the answer began with love at the center, surrounded by the following five off-shoots: comfort, attachment, inclusion, occupation, and identity. Individuals with dementia need comfort or warmth to "remain in one piece" when they may feel as though they are falling apart (Kitwood, 1997). They need to feel attachment when they so often feel as though they are in a strange place. They need to be included and involved in care and in life. They need more than simply to be occupied; they need to be involved in past and current interests and sources of fulfillment and satisfaction. Finally, people need to have an identity and their caregivers must help maintain that identity. As Kitwood stated, "To have an identity is to know who one is, in cognition and in feeling. It means having a sense of continuity with the past; and hence a 'narrative,' a story to present to others" (Kitwood, 1997). People with dementia need others to "hold their story" and to respond to them as "thou, in the uniqueness of their being" (Kitwood, 1997).

Person-Centered Care and the Culture Change Movement

The terms *person-centered care*, *person-directed care*, and even *culture change* are often used interchangeably. Although not exactly the same, they generally refer to care or a care philosophy in which a positive relationship is established that respects the person's life history and preferences, honors identity, ensures engagement in meaningful activity, and encourages an overall sense of well-being. Person-centered care can mean different things to different people in different environments. For most, it is representative of values that result in individualized care.

Brooker (2004) stated that the term *person-centered care* has its origins in the work of Carl Rogers, and that Kitwood first used the term in 1988 to distinguish a certain type of care approach from more medical and behavioral approaches to managing dementia. Kitwood used the term to bring together ideas and ways of working that emphasized communication and relationships (Brooker, 2004). Brooker added that four key components are integral to a person-centered care approach:

- Valuing people with dementia and those who care for them
- Treating people as individuals
- Looking at the world from the perspective of the person with dementia
- Providing a positive social environment in which the person with dementia can experience relative well-being (Brooker, 2004)

Downs et al. (2006) found that the person-centered care approach also has implications for care providers and family members. Rather than resulting in a loss of self, the model encourages an ongoing, evolving relationship between the care provider and the person with dementia. Care providers are no longer seen as victims, as is often the case. With adequate support and appropriate information, they will have the opportunity to redefine their relationship with the person with dementia and become enriched in the process. David Shenk (2001) stated that the care provider's challenge is to escape the medical confines of the disease and to create a new humanity within the loss.

In her book, *Design Innovations for Aging and Alzheimer's*, Elizabeth Brawley defined *culture change* as the process of moving away from a traditional nursing home model, a system that is unintentionally designed to foster dependence, to a regenerative or resident-focused model that increases the residents' autonomy and sense of control (Brawley, 2006). It is a continual process of growth and development and requires systematic change at the individual and organizational levels. The goal is to create a culture of aging that is life affirming, satisfying, humane, and meaningful (Brawley, 2006).

Brawley (2006) offered a useful summary of examples of national models for culture change that have been designed to support the self. Below are brief highlights of different care philosophies.

Resident-Directed Care. This model was designed to return control and decision making to the resident. Residents have control over their daily activities, and staff support resident decisions and share responsibility for them.

Restraint-free/Individualized Care. This model encourages and supports residents in directing their own care and returns them to familiar and comfortable routines. Physical restraints are not used, and staff are creative and compassionate when working with residents.

The Regenerative Community. This model is grounded in the belief that each resident is capable of growth and development, even if he or she is affected by a disease or disability. Residents are regarded as esteemed elders, and staff members act as community developers. Community meetings allow both staff and residents to share experiences and to make decisions.

The Eden Alternative. This model was designed to turn institutions into human habitats by bringing in plants, animals, and children. Residents have the opportunity to give and receive, and staff support variety and encourage spontaneity.

The Green House Project. This model was designed to create small, warm, smart, and green (environmentally friendly) community-based homes. Residents live in a family-style, home-like setting, and staff provide personalized care by supporting the care plan and life goals of each resident.

The Wellspring Model. This model attempts to improve resident quality of care through clinical interventions and transformation of organizational culture. Top managers assure that quality resident care is a priority, and staff support one another as they function as interdisciplinary care resource teams.

The Planetree Model. This model has the goal of personalizing, humanizing, and demystifying the healthcare system for residents and their families. Residents form *healing partnerships* with staff to support active participation in care.

More specific information on any of these models can be found through a variety of print and on-line resources. The underlying similarity that these models share is that, through innovative thinking and planning, changes have been made to ensure that the individual is the primary focus and is an instrumental contributor to the environment and to his or her own care. At the same time, this innovative thinking has resulted in organizational change in thinking and practice.

The Pioneer Network

The Pioneer Network is a notable proponent of person-centered care. A nonprofit organization, the Pioneer Network was founded in 1997 when a group of long-term care providers and advocates identified within their individual, innovative approaches a number of common principles for changing the nursing home culture. The Pioneer Network's principles stress community and relationship. They encourage care providers to know each person as a distinct individual and to place the person always before any task.

As stated on their Website (www.pioneernetwork.com), Pioneer values include the following:

- Know each person.
- Each person can and does make a difference.
- Relationship is the fundamental building block of a transformed culture.
- Respond to spirit as well as mind and body.
- Risk-taking is a normal part of life.
- Put person before the task.
- All elders are entitled to self-determination wherever they live.
- Community is the antidote to institutionalization.
- Do unto others as you would have them do unto you.
- Promote the growth and development of all.
- Shape and use the potential of the environment in all its aspects: physical, organizational, and psychosocial/spiritual.
- Practice self-examination, searching for new creativity and opportunities for doing better.
- Recognize that culture change and transformation are not destinations but a journey, always a work in progress.

The following table outlines characteristics of the traditional medical model and how actions and interactions would shift using a Pioneer model. Use this as a springboard for creative thinking about care approaches within a person-centered care culture.

Table 1.1. A Cultural Comparison: The Paradigm Shift (from the TLC in LTC of Illinois Website www.tlcinltc.org)

Traditional Medical Model	Pioneer Model
The staff provide *treatments* to *patients*.	The staff nurture the residents' human spirit in addition to meeting medical needs.
The residents follow the facility's routine.	The care setting follows residents' individual routines.
The staff floats from resident to resident.	The staff have permanent assignments.
The staff make the decisions for residents.	The residents make their own decisions.
The facility belongs to the staff.	The care setting is the residents' home.
Activities are structured and rigid.	Activities are spontaneous and available at any time.
The focus is on each department.	The focus is on the team.
The residents are known by their diagnosis.	Each resident is known as a person.

Person-Centered Language

The past decade has witnessed an exciting transformation in how we think about Alzheimer's disease (AD) and the people affected by it. In both literature and practice, the focus is beginning to shift from the disease to the *person* with the disease. Such a change takes time as well as thought and effort for practices and language to truly become more person-focused.

As mentioned before, person-centered care is based on the fundamental premise that each individual is unique and, therefore, care should be based on each person's strengths, interests, and needs. Although strides in care are being made every day, many still struggle with how to bring a person-centered philosophy to life in programs and practice, as well as how to overcome the challenges it can present. Some of those challenges, however, are often a result of falling back on old ways of thinking, acting, and speaking. What we actually do, or try to do, can be different from what we say or how we say it.

The Language of Alzheimer's Disease

An essential part of person-centered care is person-centered language. Think about some of the words that are still used to describe people with AD and their actions: *patient, victim, sufferer,* even *shell.* Their actions or behaviors are described as aggressive, agitated, inappropriate, and burdensome. These words, and others like them, are not the language of person-centered care. The words we use and our actions have a significant effect on how we think about and treat people with AD.

As you will see in Chapter Four, the current view of AD is largely negative and focuses on problematic and popular topics. This focus presents a limited, narrow view of the disease as well as of the person affected by it. Person-centered care, on the other hand, is based on respect, dignity, and possibility. To truly be centered on the person, one must always speak about and treat the person as just that—a person. It is essential, therefore, to find and use words that reflect person-centered care and that do not limit or restrict it.

The Impact of Words

Words shape thoughts and actions. They create different perspectives and form a language that impacts perceptions. Words come with *baggage* and possess universal as well as individual meanings that shape the consciousness of the people who use them (Muller & Cox Dzurec, 1993; Gayle, 1989). In addition, words can influence and lead to misconceptions and victimizations.

As illustration, the daughter of a person with Alzheimer's shared her reaction to how her father was referred to during a hospitalization. She described with much frustration how her father was variously called a victim, vegetable, and shell. "I never considered my father a shell of a human being. A shell is something lying in the garbage, like an eggshell. It's something you throw away. You don't love, care for, and respect a shell, but you do a person," she said with passion.

The power of words and language is evident when considering the effects of labeling. Labels become a permanent part of a person and help to shape his or her personal and social identity. They dehumanize the individual, limit his or her potential, and at times lead the individual to withdraw and distance him- or herself (Goffman, 1963). This dehumanization becomes apparent with AD as stages, terms, categories, and tests are developed and applied to provide some sort of uniformity to the uncertainty of the disease. The chart that follows outlines the effects of labels (top portion), as

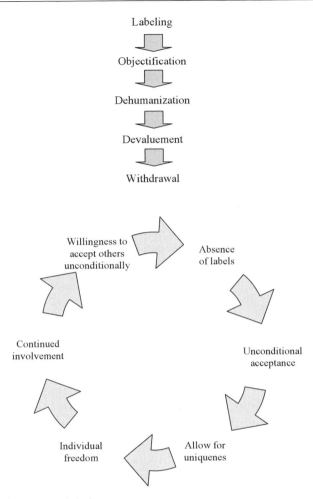

Figure 1.1. Labeling vs. not labeling

well as the possibilities that can emerge when labels do not exist (bottom portion).

This culture of negativity and use of dehumanizing words and labels is reinforced and fostered by many health care professionals. For instance, they frequently prepare families for the *difficult* road ahead or try to help by suggesting caregiving techniques that manage, control, and restrict the person with AD. These professionals' interventions are often one dimensional and focus only on the immediate needs of the caregiver. In addition, health care professionals often try to apply a medical structure to an ambiguous and, at times, nonmedical experience.

The medical model of dementia care, sometimes called the *illness model*, focuses on abnormalities in the structure and function of body organs that lead to disease. The medical view of dementia is narrow and sometimes ignores social forces that affect the definition, development, and progression of dementia. Sociologist Karen Lyman proposed a shift in how the disease is considered to include a more social perspective. This shift includes social factors, nonmedical terminology, and recognition of the individual (Lyman, 1993).

Recognizing the individual, or the person, is difficult with so much negativity and focus on abnormalities and problems. If an individual is continually invalidated and objectified, he or she can lose more and more vital contact with others, which can be considered a significant part of personhood. We must move beyond losses and begin to recognize and support strengths and abilities. As one family member said, "He can still do a lot of things if we'd take the time to find them out and then just let him do them the best he can."

The clinical focus, which currently looks only at problems, should also assess remaining strengths, positive functions, and individual characteristics (Harrison, 1993). Many believe that by recognizing the strengths and working with the remaining abilities of people with AD, we can improve the care as well as the disease experience. However, strengths can be difficult to recognize within the context of the existing descriptions of this disease.

A technique called *reframing* can be used to help people recognize the positive aspects of situations that were previously viewed as only negative. Reframing has been defined as "thinking about things in a different way; relabeling and redefining behavior, or finding the 'positive connotation' of a behavior or situation" (Pesut, 1991, p. 10). By reframing a symptom, we can understand it as serving a positive function, and, in a sense, every experience and every behavior is appropriate given some context, some frame (Bandler & Grinder, 1982; Benson, Long & Sporakowski, 1992). Once a situation has been reframed into a more positive context, more choices become available for coping with the challenges that may arise. When additional options become available, often the tensions and pressures that are associated with seemingly hopeless or burdensome situations are alleviated and alternatives become apparent (Hulnick & Hulnick, 1989). Reframing is not about making the disease positive, but rather describing things in a different way to open our minds to new ways of thinking and acting.

The impact of our descriptions is powerful. Our words shape perceptions, experiences, and approaches to caregiving. Less negative and more positive alternatives must begin to be used to describe AD. The use of positive alternatives, such as reframing, can help people construct their beliefs based on a more encompassing or balanced view. Families and other caregivers can form new opinions of how to approach the disease when they are introduced to other ways of looking at experiences besides a largely negative view. Their approaches to caregiving will then be more positive, as will their overall experience of the disease. They then can begin to recognize the opportunities for growth and personal development rather than focusing on loss, decline, and the burden of caregiving. Although feelings associated with loss and burden are real, they are not all that people feel throughout the disease process.

In addition, families and other caregivers can begin to recognize how their actions affect the behaviors of the person with AD. If they develop a more person-centered view of the disease, individual differences and characteristics can more readily be recognized and accepted and, as a result, the care experience for the person with AD can be more beneficial. Programs and interactions can acknowledge strengths and abilities and be designed to support them.

The impact of language on perception and behavior is immense. If people become more aware of words, thoughts, and behaviors, Alzheimer care and interactions may improve dramatically. Individuals must begin to recognize the weight words bear and how those words shape perceptions, experiences, and approaches to care. Families should not have to filter out negativity to *survive* and *function*. We must rethink our descriptions and offer less negative alternatives to the common dismal words and labels used to describe AD, the individuals who experience it, and our interactions with them. Using person-centered language is the first step in embracing a person-centered philosophy of caring.

Caring and Person-Centered Care

The book *Rethinking Alzheimer's Care* explores the concept of caring in some detail with the leadership of Dorothy Seman (Fazio, Seman & Stansell, 1999). Since a caring relationship is fundamental to person-centered care, it may be helpful to highlight some of the key elements of that discussion.

Caring has been described as a moral ideal that rests within a person. This ideal is reflected in one's personal commitment to relate to others in a way that preserves dignity and restores humanity. This way of relating does not make the person who is receiving care feel as though he or she is an object (Watson, 1988). It is an intentional and interpersonal process with an underlying respect for personal worth. Kristen Swanson-Kaufman (1986) defined caring as a nurturing way of relating to another valued person with whom one feels a personal sense of commitment and responsibility. Through her nursing research she observed five processes that she identified as examples of caring: maintaining belief, knowing, being with, doing for, and enabling.

Maintaining belief is conveying to the person that he or she has the capacity to get through events or transitions and to face a future with meaning.

Knowing is trying to understand an event as it has meaning in the life of the person.

Being with is conveying the feeling of being emotionally present to the person.

Doing for is giving assistance to the individual in the performance of those activities that the person would perform unaided if he or she had the necessary strength, will, or knowledge to do so.

Enabling is facilitating the individual's passage through life transitions and unfamiliar events.

Although not specifically developed in relation to people with AD, these five processes can help us to understand how caring can take place with persons with AD across all care settings.

Callahan (2001) described caring in somewhat different terms but with similar intent. Caring

- Focuses on the needs of the recipient
- Is offered regardless of the probability that the recipient will recover what he or she has lost
- Aims at psychological and spiritual needs as well as purely physical ones
- Addresses both the general and specific needs of recipients
- Is relational
- Focuses primarily on alleviating suffering

Callahan also discussed four general levels of caring that are appropriate to everyone: cognitive, feeling and emotion, values, and relational. Caring is not something we do apart from our everyday interactions; it is incorporated into each and every human exchange in which we engage.

Caring for the Person, Not the Disease

A key element of a person-centered caring relationship is *caring for the person, not the disease.* There is often a tendency for caregivers to relate exclusively or primarily to an individual with a disease only in terms of his or her disease. In a sense, the person is not engaged as the unique human being he or she is, but in terms of the symptoms he or she displays. This diminishes the individual's potential and limits the many opportunities to engage on a deeper, more gratifying level of exchange with him or her. Throughout the disease process, individuals with dementia still respond in quite predictable ways to positive and negative human exchanges. As Dr. William Osler stated, "It is much more important to know what sort of a patient has a disease than what sort of disease a patient has." By striving to look beyond the symptoms to the full human being, we discover many opportunities to connect with that individual in a variety of ways. Although caring for a person is more of an overall philosophy rather than a specific action, starting a conversation with a simple, "How are you feeling today?" or "How has your day been so far?" can allow you to connect with the person and show that you care.

Beyond Simply Providing Care

Caring also involves *more than simply providing care.* A caring culture should encourage a deeper level of personal care and commitment that cannot be outlined in any job description. In any care setting, there are many opportunities to provide comfort, share daily joys and sorrows, and interact in authentic ways that acknowledge that the person is much more than a resident, patient, or participant. The person is a unique individual with needs and feelings of his or her own. He or she has much to offer and to give, if we are open to the possibilities. We can invite a deeper level of involvement that opens doors to a rich and more satisfying relationship that can be of mutual benefit. For instance, weaving into a conversation a cherished fact about the person's life, a specific preference, or a significant event can let the person know that you are interested in and care about him or her. At the same time, asking the person for his or her opinion about a topic can tell the person that you value his or her perspective.

Focus on Connecting, Not Correcting

Person-centered care also *shifts the focus from correcting to connecting.* Having dementia often affects one's ability to remember and/or to express specific facts about particular roles and relationships. However, the majority of individuals with dementia have a great capacity for engaging in gratifying human interactions. This can be discovered when others look carefully, are attentive to possibilities, and approach the person in an open, accepting, and giving way.

In focusing on the quality of the relationship and not on a particular task to be done as part of daily care, it is important to evaluate the ways in which act with persons with AD in everyday situations. Specific facts are insignificant and the underlying intent, feeling, or meaning are much more important. Caregivers commonly use language and behavior that focus on correcting the individual with dementia. Warnings and directives that are filled with *shoulds* and *don'ts* are frequently used. Often the facial expression, body language, and tone of voice of the caregiver are very firm, abrupt, or stern, which can convey a message of control that may be perceived as quite discomforting, if not outright threatening, to a person with AD.

In shifting the focus to caring about the person, the ways we provide care also need to change. The entire framework of communication needs to be modified in ways that are more positive and affirming and that focus on *connecting and not correcting.* This change is not merely one of using new words, but rather reconsidering a whole new approach that puts the person with AD, and our relationship with him or her, at the heart of the communication. Instead of saying, "Don't go there," "Don't touch that," you might step back and think about ways to accomplish the same goals without demeaning or reducing the person. For example, "Could you help me?" or "Would you come this way?" are alternatives that help to refocus a person with AD, while at the same time engage and invite, not demean and control. They are ways to connect rather than to correct.

Listening for Meaning

Caring also involves *listening for meaning.* Often the quietly spoken comments of persons with dementia go unheard by the caregiver, and even go unshared with the rest of the staff. An individual with AD may say something that does not exactly fit into the conversation at the time, or that may take a bit of discussion to understand the meaning. These types of comments can be viewed as gifts to be recognized and appreciated in the here and now, and to learn from. Even the negative comments can help, by giving us a window into how the person who is receiving our care feels about it. Taken together, they can help us do more of some things and less of others. They can help us develop more sensitive and caring approaches.

Often comments carry complex meanings that give us insight into the way individuals are thinking and feeling about their life and about what is happening to them. These comments can help us to understand their needs and how we can assist them and can offer guidance for providing the right kind of support and care throughout the course of the illness. A favorite example of listening for meaning is a man being assisted with putting on his jacket who said, in a rather quick manner, "Who do you think I am? Houdini?" (meaning, "Slow down, I'm going as fast as I can"). Although he did not actually say to slow down, it was clear what he was trying to get across, or the meaning behind his words.

By recognizing and understanding verbal and nonverbal responses from the person being cared for, caregivers can measure whether their care approach is succeeding and can modify the approach based on the feedback. Staff should not measure success only by the completion of a task, such as the number of baths provided or meals served, but rather by how the person being cared for feels about the care he or she is receiving. With a greater awareness of facial expressions, body language, and verbal and nonverbal language (reading between the lines), caregivers can have greater insight into how the person experienced the care that was provided. In other words, success must not be limited to counting up what was done, but should include how it felt to the persons being cared for. By tuning into feedback, staff can change the care approach so that the experience can feel safer, more enjoyable, and more gratifying and meaningful for the person with dementia as well as for the staff member.

Communicate Caring in Everyday Care

It is also important to *communicate caring in our everyday care*. Once we commit to *caring for* and not just *taking care of* persons with dementia, we can and must think about ways that caring can be woven into our daily encounters. This care approach requires us to examine the way we interact throughout the day with the person in our care. It may help to ask ourselves how we would react to the care if our roles were reversed. Would I be satisfied to be on the receiving end of the care I provide? Am I open to really observing and listening and to not focusing exclusively on my agenda of what tasks need to be done? Am I flexible enough to change my attitudes and behavior if they seem to interfere with rather than support the quality of life of the person I'm caring for? Sometimes a simple pat on the back, rub on the arm, smile, or handshake can show that you care, especially when providing everyday care.

Finally, we must consider how to *foster a caring community*. Healthy adult relationships are usually described in terms of their mutuality and reciprocity, as well as in the ease of give and take in everyday life. This kind of caring culture helps the care recipient feel and experience care in different ways. The person being cared for is not just being helped, but is also able to help others, to give. He or she is part of a caring community. There are many opportunities to help a person with AD maintain the continuity of life-long roles and to achieve the satisfaction of contributing to others in diverse ways as the person had done throughout his or her life. For example, a teacher may enjoy being part of a children's group, an office worker may want to help stuff envelopes for a community organization, a homemaker may like to help set a table for lunch, or a plumber may find satisfaction in helping unclog a sink.

Core Values in Providing Person-Centered Care

In *Rethinking Alzheimer's Care*, the following core values in providing care were introduced (Fazio, Seman & Stansell, 1999). In providing person-centered care that maintains the self, it is important to approach every relationship and interaction with these core values in mind.

Everyone Should Be Treated with Dignity and Respect

It is dismaying that this statement still needs to be said, but it does. It seems so fundamental. My hope is that one day we will no longer need to say it. People with dementia should be treated like people, like human beings, and with dignity and respect in every situation.

Relate to the Person, not the Disease or Symptoms

It is so important to relate to the person with AD, not to the disease itself. In so many situations, a person with dementia is defined by the symptoms of the disease, and who he or she has been for a lifetime is ignored. The disease should become another part of who the person is, not solely who the person is. We must find ways to relate to the person with the disease and to the lifelong self. Kitwood asserted that we must recognize the *full humanity* of people with dementia. It is not acceptable to speak of a person with dementia, but rather a *person* with dementia (Kitwood, 1997).

Control Issues Do Not Exist

As care providers, we do not always need to be in control of the situation. Granted, people need to be kept safe and secure and out of harm's way, but not through controlling and restrictive methods. When faced with a challenging situation, it is important to stop and ask, "What if this were to play out differently than I had planned, would it really matter?"

Autonomy Is More than Choices

People with dementia need to be involved in making choices, but they also can be a part of making decisions, when appropriate. These can be small decisions, such as planning a day, or large decisions, such as planning for the future. Autonomy is about feeling in control of one's actions and situations. We must find ways to allow individuals to feel in control and involved.

Dementia Is More than Loss and Decline—People Retain Skills

There is unquestionably loss and decline associated with AD, but that is not all there is. People with dementia have retained skills and abilities, but often they need others to help maintain or support them. Use of those retained skills is fundamental to the preservation of self. Interactions with and programs for people with AD must be based on strengths and abilities, not on loss and inability.

To Facilitate the Use of Retained Skills, One Must Compensate for Losses

In order for a person to be successful, he or she needs to be in a situation, environment, or relationship that allows him or her to succeed. A person needs to be in a supportive relationship and environment that compensates for his or her losses and that allows him or her to use retained skills. This might be as simple as the caregiver initiating the use of those skills (e.g., demonstrating brushing hair or putting on shoes), or as involved as creating a supportive environment that allows for success (e.g., laying out the necessary articles of clothing for an outfit).

Basic Human Needs Are the Same for Everyone

People with dementia are human beings and have the same needs as everyone else. In addition to basic care needs, people with dementia need to feel loved, to express their emotions, to be successful, and to have the opportunity to grow and evolve. As stated earlier, caring goes beyond providing basic care.

Getting to Know the Person and the Self: An Essential First Step

Unlike family members who have a history with the individual, care professionals typically do not know the person until he or she comes into their care. The information they do know often comes from an initial assessment, from other staff members, or hopefully from the person and his or her family. There are an abundance of tools to assess an individual with AD. The goal here is not to create another tool. Instead, beyond the usual assessments, there are additional areas to consider when getting to know a person with AD. It is important to spend time finding out who the person is and who he or she has been throughout his or her life. It is essential to get to know a person's lifelong self and not just who he or she is in relation to the disease's symptoms.

Rethinking Alzheimer's Care identified several different areas to consider during assessments, including:

- Core identity
- Social history
- Life interests
- Communication
- Way of relating to others
- Cognitive status/judgment
- Responsiveness to the environment
- Physical functional capacity
- Health

There are many other categories that can be added to the list. Whichever areas are explored, it is important to find out the essence of the individual— who the person is and what he or she values. It is essential to understand how the person has lived his or her life, including skills, interests, support systems, and how the individual has derived meaning in his or her life. At the same time, it is important to find out about a person's current essence, including preferences, how he or she communicates, what he or she might find to be upsetting, and his or her functional abilities.

SELF-Portrait—The *Essence* of Frances

Frances has always been a very passionate person. She has always been known for her ability to tell you what she thinks. Despite her declining verbal abilities, she is still very expressive and tries to get her message across to others. She frequently claps her hands together when pleased or excited, and will often clutch your arm when alarmed or upset. Having grown up near a national park, Frances loves nature and the outdoors. Nowadays, she enjoys a walk in the garden and watching the birds and squirrels through the window. Frances likes to be involved in things but often does not initiate her participation. She responds well to encouragement, but if rushed she will refuse to do anything.

Learning about how an individual would prefer to spend his or her day is also important. Think about how you spend a typical day—the ebb and flow of the day, the natural rhythm and the choices that you make. The choices that we make and the flow of our typical day are representative of and impact who we are, our self. Similarly, for a person with AD, it is important to find out from the individual and from family members what a typical day would look like. The typical day should not have to change so drastically when a person with AD enters a new living environment. Finding ways to support those typical days is then the necessary next step.

SELF-Portrait—John's Typical Day

John grew up on a farm and worked in the field for most of his life. His mornings started very early, before the sun came up. Before he went to work, John would enjoy a strong cup of coffee in the silence of his kitchen. After working for several hours, he would come back to the house for a break and for a big home-cooked breakfast that his wife would prepare for him. John would work a few more hours outdoors in the fields, and then enjoy a light lunch while reading the newspaper. Afternoons often included odd jobs around the farm, transporting goods, or running errands in town. John's wife always cooked a big dinner, and evenings mostly consisted of watching television, listening to the radio, or sitting on the front porch and looking at the evening stars. These daily patterns are still very important and meaningful to John.

Individuals have and need various types of relationships with a variety of different people. It is important to learn about the types of relationships a person has had throughout his or her life as well as the meanings he or she attaches to them. These relationships include relationships with him- or herself, with family and friends, with a spiritual world or entity, and with the broader community. It is important to have a good understanding of the meaning and importance of the relationships an individual has had throughout his or her life.

SELF-Portrait—Katherine's Relationships

Katherine's family has always been the most important thing in her life. Even as a child, she used to always talk about being a wife and a mother, and she spent countless hours playing house with her friends. Katherine was an only child, and adored her parents. She married her childhood sweetheart, Don, and had a special connection with him. They were best friends and shared everything with one another. Their friends and family say they never saw them have a fight or be disrespectful to each other in any way. Katherine's three children mean everything to her. Being all girls, Katherine and her children often seemed more like close friends. She has two grandchildren, who she often refers to as "little angels." Friends are also important to Katherine, as she considers them extensions of her family. She has many lifelong friends with whom she has kept in touch over the years. Others know her as a good friend and a very caring person.

To truly provide a person-centered approach to care and to maintain self-hood, caregivers must find out who the person has been throughout his or her life, not only who the person is now. One approach to getting to know the whole person can be found in wellness and holistic literature, which often discusses the following six domains of selfhood that make up a person:

- Physical
- Social
- Emotional
- Intellectual
- Spiritual
- Vocational, professional, or occupational

Thinking about the self in a holistic framework (see Figure 1.2) is an important way to remind us about the many different aspects of a person and to challenge us to broaden our perspective. Caregivers can assess a person with AD in each area and can make adjustments to the care approach to maintain the *wellness* of the person in each of the six areas. The importance of each domain varies from individual to individual.

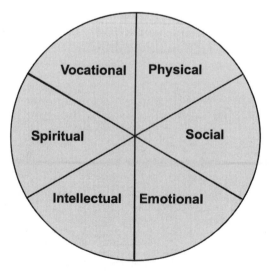

Figure 1.2. Domains of Self

Another useful approach to getting to know the whole person is to use the attribute categories outlined by Sabat and Collins (1999), which are expanded upon in the research described in Chapter Four. You can look at these categories as representative aspects of a person. They include:

- Physical traits
- Personal characteristics and qualities
- Familial
- Vocational or professional
- Educational
- Talents, hobbies and interests
- Attitudes and beliefs

For the six domains of self and the attribute categories, it is important to think about how well you know the people with dementia you are caring for in relation to each of the areas. It is also important to think about who you can ask or where you can go to find out more about the individual in relation to the areas.

It is also important to glean information from a variety of sources and at different times throughout the person's illness. Be sure to begin with the person with dementia. Ask the person what he or she thinks is the best way for

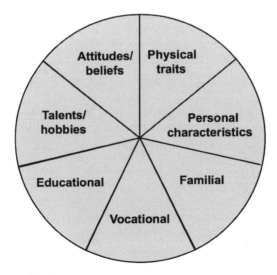

Figure 1.3. Attributes of Self

a caregiver to get to know him or her. Ask what he or she thinks the caregiver should do with the information he or she has given about his or her life. Also, consider developing an *I-assessment,* which would allow the individual to construct *I* statements (e.g., "I like to . . ."). Keep in mind that many factors, such as confusion or mood, time restraints, and an inappropriate assessment tool, can influence the accuracy of the information obtained through an assessment. Therefore, you may need to talk on an ongoing basis rather than just once and to complete an assessment over time. Besides speaking with the person with dementia, it is essential to speak with other caregivers as well as relatives, friends, and colleagues. Direct observation is also key. It is important to get to know the person through a variety of ways and at a variety of times. Remember that the overall goal is not only to focus on the past or the present, but also on a combination of both and also on how they can work together to allow for interactions and activities that promote selfhood.

The above examples are meant to illustrate ways we can unconventionally (beyond typical assessment tools) get to know a person with AD and find out more about the self. The process is less important than the outcome: getting to know who the person is so that we can foster interactions and create programs that support the individual and that maintain the individual's selfhood. It is important that you find a tool or process that works best for you and for your community. It is also important to find ways to share what you learn with others. You may want to put together a life-story book, share stories of individuals at team meetings, or develop an ongoing life-story project. Another example is to include a "Did you know" exercise in team meetings, where caregivers share a fact about an individual they are caring for (e.g., "Did you know that Marion was a competitive ice-skater?"). Caregivers can discuss how certain facts about the individuals they are caring for can be incorporated into programs and interactions. It is essential that you find ways for the stories to live on and to continue to develop. Finally, it is most important to move from assessment to action, to develop a plan that incorporates what you know into daily interactions and care. These tools and processes will be discussed in more detail in the chapters in Section II.

Closing

There are many tenets of person-centered care that are equivalent to care that maintains the self. The self is the core of the person. Each caregiver or care facility must first look at individual and organizational values and make sure these reflect a person-centered focus. These values influence how each person or organization thinks about and approaches care and interactions. Thinking about care in a person-centered framework is the first step in developing a community that supports and maintains the self. Before discussing specific care practices, however, it may be helpful to understand some of the theory and research related to the self and Alzheimer's care.

PROVIDING CARE THAT AFFIRMS PERSONHOOD

Kitwood (1997) described components of interpersonal care that affirm personhood. Think about the people you care for. Are your care and interactions reflective of these components? If not, what can you do differently to provide care in a way that is reflective of these personhood-affirming components?

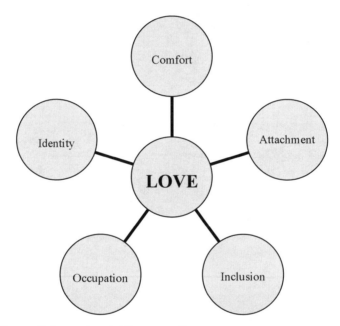

Figure 1.4. Kitwood's Personhood Affirmation Components

SELF-Reflection

USING NEW WORDS TO DESCRIBE ALZHEIMER'S DISEASE AND THE PERSON

Think about some negative words that are used to talk about Alzheimer's disease or to refer to the person with the disease and his or her symptoms or behaviors. Make a list of those words on the left-hand side of a page. On the right-hand side, make another list of alternative or less negative words that correspond with those you identified. How do you think perceptions and approaches to care and interactions might change if the negative words were viewed differently? How would self or personhood be affected?

Examples:

Common negative word	Alternative, less negative
Victim, sufferer	Person, individual
Agitated	Energetic
Problem behavior	Challenging behavior
Aggressive	Passionate
Short attention span	Curious

SELF-Reflection

GETTING TO KNOW A PERSON THROUGH ASSESSMENT—A CHECKLIST

Rather than creating another assessment tool, this checklist will help you to review your current assessment tools. Consider your current ways of finding out who a person is and who the person has been throughout his or her life. Are you gaining enough information to know a person in each of these areas? Are you talking to enough people to really get to know who the person is?

___ Core identity

___ Family history, social and cultural history, vocational or occupational history

___ Life interests

___ Communication, ways of relating, responsiveness to environment

___ Cognitive status, health, physical functional capacity

___ Relationships

___ Strengths, needs and abilities

___ Typical day

GETTING TO KNOW THE ENTIRE SELF AND CREATING A
PERSON-CENTERED PLAN

Choose one of the two models illustrated below. Think about the person and how to get to know him or her in the areas identified in each model. Find out who he or she has been and who he or she is now. Ask him or her and others, such as family and friends. Find out about the person's lifelong and current self. Begin to think about how activities and interactions can be built to support and maintain all of these aspects of self and to reflect both the lifelong and current self.

Domains of Self

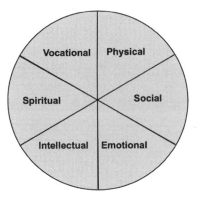

Attributes of Self
(Explained in more detail in Chapter 4)

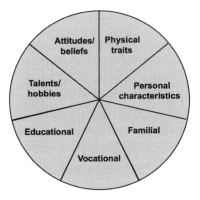

CHAPTER TWO

OVERVIEW OF SELF

Self is the knowledge, feelings, and attitudes we have about our own being as unique, functioning individuals.

Lemme (1999)

Given a disease process that can affect a person's ability to express his or her identity, it is not surprising that people generally assume that a person with moderate to advanced Alzheimer's disease (AD) is no longer self-aware. But what is this *self* of which a person is (or is not) aware? Philosophers, psychologists, sociologists, writers, and many others have struggled with this question throughout human history; that is, how to describe, understand, or quantify one's sense of unique awareness or identity. This chapter summarizes some of the most useful theories about the self as a foundation for understanding how to recognize and acknowledge the enduring self in people with dementia.

Maintaining the self in people with Alzheimer's begins with an understanding of the multidimensional nature of the self and how it likely develops from childhood through adulthood. It is helpful to look at some theories of early development in childhood because it is here that self-awareness can be observed to begin and where it operates at its simplest level. The challenges of recognizing and assessing self-awareness in young children who have limited language and communication skills can be similar for people with dementia. Unlike children, however, people with dementia have identities formed by the experiences of a lifetime. In order to appreciate the level of self-awareness that persists throughout the course of AD, it is therefore also necessary to examine what is known about the more complex adult self. The self, for example, does not exist in a vacuum, but is influenced—some even say is formed—by interactions with other people and with the environment, and it is in this context that caregivers may have the greatest opportunity for supporting the self in Alzheimer's care.

Finally, researchers have demonstrated that each person's identity evolves over time, adapting to many changes, particularly to losses in old age. There is surprising resilience and adaptability in the aging self, which is important to realize in considering the effects of any late-life disease, including AD. This chapter provides a background that is essential to understanding the self in AD.

Definitions of *Self* and Theories of Early Development

Self is a key construct in psychology as well as other disciplines. However, the way *self* is defined and used differs among theorists and fields of study. From an early philosophical point of view, John Locke (1689) describes the self as the agent responsible for the thoughts and actions of an individual to which they are ascribed. He maintained that the self endures through time, and that the thoughts and actions at different moments of time may pertain to the same self. From a psychological perspective, the self generally refers to the conscious, reflective personality of an individual. Lemme (1999) described the self as the knowledge, feelings, and attitudes we have about our own being as unique, functioning individuals.

Other terms often are used interchangeably for *self*, such as *self-knowledge*, *self-awareness*, *self-consciousness*, or *identity*. Although very similar, there are some distinct differences among them. *Self-knowledge* commonly refers to knowledge of one's particular mental states, including one's beliefs, desires, and sensations. *Self-awareness* refers to the explicit understanding that one exists as an individual, separate from other people and with private thoughts. *Self-consciousness* refers to the personal understanding of the very core of one's own identity (Newman & Newman, 1995).

Identity is a broader term used in the social sciences to refer to an individual's comprehension of him- or herself as a discrete, separate entity (Newman & Newman, 1995). Identity is a sense of who one is, where one is going in life, and how one fits into society (Shaffer, 2002). Newman and Newman (1995) stated that the structure of identity has two components: content and evaluation, similar to the psychological self. Content (what one thinks about, values, and believes in, and the traits or characteristics by which one is recognized and known by others) may be further divided into the private self and the public self. The private self, often described as a sense of self, refers to one's inner uniqueness and unity, a subjective experience of being the originator of one's thoughts and actions and of being self-reflective. The elements of public self include the many roles a person plays and the expectations of others. The second structural component of identity, evaluation, refers to the capacity for self-reflection and the awareness of self.

References to the self can be seen in the early writings of William James, the father of psychology. In *The Principles of Psychology*, James (1950) devoted significant attention to the concept of self and described a distinction between two selves. He defined the *categorical self*, or the *me*, as an object with specific traits, characteristics, likes, and dislikes and the *subjective self*, or the *I*, as reflected in the ongoing stream of consciousness, the central knower or experiencer.

Over the years, many other researchers have expanded upon the definitions of self discussed above and have formulated theories of their own, all of which include distinctions between or the duality of *I* and *me* (Lewis, 1991; Lewis & Brookes-Gunn, 1979; Nelson, 2001; Povinelli, 1995). Lewis and Brookes-Gunn (1979) defined the duality of self as the existential self and the categorical self. Lewis (1991) expanded upon this distinction and suggested that when attention is directed inward, we focus on ourselves and we are the objects of our own consciousness, or what he called objective self-awareness (me-self). When attention is directed away from us, we are the subject of the consciousness that is directed toward external objects, or what he referred to as subjective self-awareness (I-self).

In a related theory, Povinelli (1995; 2001) maintained that the self continues to develop from an initial system of self-representations that is largely restricted in the here and now (the present self) to a later system that is capable of temporal differentiation (the proper self). Other developmental psychologists have described how the self is crafted through the construction of narratives that provide the basis for autobiographical memory (Harter, 1999). Nelson (2001) stated that an indication of a sense of self can be gleaned from language, most specifically late in the second year or early in the third year, when children begin using personal pronouns. Similarly, Fivush (2001) argued that one critical aspect of the development of a sense of self that is continuous in time is the construction of an autobiographical self, a self based on the specific experiences the individual recalls. In AD, caregivers notice changes in this type of self and often conclude that the self no longer exists. However, as we will discuss in Chapter Four, these changes may have more to do with the inability to independently construct and communicate the autobiographical self than with its absence.

Researchers have also addressed the continued development of self and its components throughout the life course. James (1950) described the self as having three major multidimensional and hierarchical constituents: the material self, the social self, and the spiritual self. Giarrusso, Mabry, and Bengston (2001) described the self as made up of three basic components: the cognitive (the content of who we are), the affective (the feelings about who we are), and the conative (our actions on the basis of our self-perceptions). Other researchers have described the self as both a cognitive and social construction, related to developmental stages (Harter, 1999), and how new dimensions are added in adolescence, adulthood, and older adulthood (Lemme, 1999).

Social Construction of the Self

Many researchers have theorized and examined how social interactions shape and support the self (Harter, 1999; Pelham & Hetts, 1999; Stetsenko & Arievitch, 1997; Turner & Onorato, 1999). Pelham and Hetts (1999) posited that a person's self concept is a product of his or her interactions and identifications with other people. Turner and Onorato (1999) stated:

> The social self is a looking glass self, a function of how people appear and are reacted to by "others" (individuals, groups, society, the generalized other). The looking glass self is a metaphor for the idea that the individual sees (acquires) self in the "reflected appraisals" of others. (p. 14)

The authors found that others provide social reflections of the self that, when internalized, make self-awareness reflexive, provide social identities, and enable participation in a world with shared symbolic meanings:

> The self is social, therefore, insofar as it projects public identities in social interaction, enacts social roles and norms, is presented to and perceived by others, is shaped by their expectations, and contains the internalized reactions, expectations, and judgments of others. (p. 14)

A fundamental concept here is the idea that the self is a social product that is created and validated by an individual's interaction with significant others (Harter, 1999). In this theory, called symbolic interactionism, the self is viewed as a social construction, which is crafted through linguistic exchanges, or symbolic interactions, with others (Harter, 1999). Many theorists agree with this concept. In his early writings, Cooley (1902) described his belief that significant others constituted a social mirror into which the person gazes to gain the opinions toward the self. These opinions are then incorporated into one's sense of self. There is significant evidence, through the research of people such as Kitwood (1997), that people with dementia react to such opinions and expectations.

Other early researchers stressed the importance of social influence on the self. Mead (1925) found that the individual comes to adopt the generalized perspective of a group of significant others who share a particular societal perspective of the self. Baldwin (1897) argued that the construction of self was a very social and dialectical or communicative process between the self and another person. Goffman (1959) suggested that individuals have multiple selves and that one's personal identity persists behind the publicly presented repertoire of one's personae. Harter (1999) summarized several themes across these theorists and concluded that the role of opinions of others is paramount in shaping the concept of self through social interaction, and that the individual assimilates the self-attributes originally encouraged or identified by others into his or her habitual sense of self. In short, the self is influenced by other people, which is the most critical message for people who are providing dementia care.

Measurements of Self

Some ways of measuring an awareness of self in people with dementia have evolved from techniques used to measure awareness of self in young, pre-verbal children. Visual self-recognition has been used to assess knowledge of self before words and as a useful indicator of underlying self-awareness (Lewis & Brooks-Gunn, 1979; Ross, 1992). Many researchers have used the ability of 18- to 24-month-old children to recognize themselves in mirrors as evidence of a developed self-concept (Brooks-Gunn & Lewis, 1984; Howe & Courage, 1993). In a related approach, Povinelli (2001) studied delayed or re-representations in which he related past instances of self to the present state by showing children representations of previous visual instances of themselves in videotapes and photographs.

Several researchers have examined the use of language and autobio-graphical memory as indicators of self in early childhood (Fivush, 2001; Nelson, 2001). Other researchers have discussed autobiographical memory and its relation to self-awareness in adolescents and adults (Addis & Tip-pett, 2004; Gil et al., 2001). Gil et al. (2001) described self-awareness as the consciousness of one's own history, of one's autobiography. Addis and Tippett (2004) posited that autobiographical memory contributes to trait self-knowledge (self-identifications and perceptions of oneself) and to self-narratives (stories about oneself, one's life and experiences), enabling the integration of past and present selves and contributing to the sense of continuity of identity. Measures such as the Tennessee Self Concept Scale have focused on self-knowledge, and measures such as the Twenty Statements Test have focused on narrative identity (Addis & Tippett, 2004).

Another approach to measuring the self is to look at conversation and discourse, exploring the use of language to represent the self (Davis & Harre, 1990; Harre, 1991). Harre (1987) suggested that the inner centeredness we call *the self* is the result of an organizational process driven by grammatical models:

> I believe we organize our experience in such a way that that experience can be reported, commented on, etc. within the linguistic resources we possess, themselves adjusted to the expression and maintenance of our local moral order. (p. 51)

Keenan et al. (2003) added that the use of personal pronouns in adults reveals a heightened sense of self-awareness.

Researchers have also examined self-awareness and the continued development of self through adolescence and adulthood (Damon & Hart, 1982; Harter, 1988). Many researchers studying this topic have used the common practice of self-report or self-evaluation tools to examine different aspects of self, including self-esteem, self-efficacy, and self-concept (Brinthaupt & Lipka, 1992; Byrne 1996). Many of these studies that have taken a self-evaluation approach explored only the affective component of self, or one's beliefs or thoughts about things. (Giarrusso, Mabry & Bengston, 2001). Markova (1987) suggested the need for studies that explore other components of self and that examine both the structure (relatively stable nature) and process (changing nature) of self. For my work related to the persistence of identity in people with dementia, I chose to use both language (self-knowledge) and self-recognition as the basis for measuring self-awareness, or the persistence of self (see Chapter Four). I found that this approach also measured the dual nature of the self—both personal and social identities.

Self-Concept, Identity, and the Evolving Self through Adulthood

The self-concept reflects the knowledge and beliefs about ourselves. It serves as a mental framework on which we organize information about ourselves and affects our perception and processing of information. It is hierarchical and dynamic and subject to revision and alteration (Lemme, 1999. James (1950) posited that people have different self-concepts, often described in a hierarchy, with the abstract or consistent self-concept being at the top while concepts related to particular situations and contexts branch out from it. He argued that the degree of similarity and level of organization among different self-concepts would vary from person to person in importance and pervasiveness. He added that changes in roles or developmental tasks may necessitate a reorganization of the hierarchy. Therefore, the current self-concept is in essence a working self-concept subject to modification and change throughout life (Schaie & Willis, 1996).

The Creation, Re-creation, and Maintenance of Self

Many researchers are understanding more about the important ways in which identity and the creation of self continue to develop through adulthood. Cavanuagh and Blanchard-Fields (2002) discussed Dan McAdams' beliefs that a person's sense of identity is based on a story of how the person came into being, where the person has been, where he or she is going, and who he or she will become. They argue that people create a life story that is an internalized narrative with a beginning, middle, and anticipated ending. It is created and revised throughout adulthood as people change and as changing environments place different demands on people. According to Cavanaugh and Blanchard-Fields, people begin forming their life story in late adolescence and early adulthood.

Cavanaugh and Blanchard-Fields (2002) also discussed Whitbourne's beliefs that people build on their own conceptions of how their lives should proceed. Whitbourne believes that people have a life-span construct, a unified sense of their past, present, and future. The components of the life-span construct are the scenario, or expectations of the future, and the life story, or a personal narrative history. Whitbourne integrates Piaget's concepts of assimilation and accommodation, or how awareness of the outside world is internalized, to explain how people's identity changes over time. Family and work are considered two major sources of identity. These areas are also important aspects of identity for people with AD. Knowing these important and individual aspects of self allows the caregiver to personalize communications and reinforce a continued sense of self.

In short, identity is created and recreated over time as a person progresses through life. The structure and meaning of one's identity is established as experiences are layered on one another and are reflected upon, evaluated, adjusted to, and incorporated. Identity is built around themes without regard to time, as past experiences are symbolically connected with one another to have meaning for the individual (Lemme, 1999). Sharon Kaufman suggested that the construction of self is an ongoing process (Lemme, 1999). Older people's identities are rooted in lifelong personal experience, and meanings are continually reinterpreted with new circumstances. A person selects events from his or her past to structure and restructure his or her identity. There is a continual creation of the self through the ongoing interpretation of past experience, structural factors, values, and current context. Hazel MacRae supported Kaufman's idea of an ageless self, and maintained that there is a core of *real me* that continues despite physical and social change (Lemme, 1999). Continuity of familiar settings, roles, and relationships contributes to stability in the sense of self over time.

Adaptation and the Self in Older Adults

Some researchers have examined how older people, faced with losses in many domains, maintain a positive sense of well-being. Lemme (1999) discussed McRae's belief that successful adaptation takes place when individuals symbolically connect meaningful past experiences with current circumstances. *Adaptation* is the process by which a person creates meaning, organizes the past, explains events, and communicates with others. Baltes and Baltes (1990) described a model of adaptation called selective optimization with compensation (SOC), which basically helps us understand why older people who are faced with losses in many domains of their lives are able to maintain a positive sense of self. The model suggests that when individuals encounter losses, such as those associated with aging, they select the most important goals and focus their efforts on optimizing performance in these areas while withdrawing from less important activities. Older adults generally adjust to losses. They continue to interpret their participation in the social world. By looking at themes that emerge from stories, we can see how people not only cope with losses, but how they create new meaning as they reformulate and build viable selves.

Some researchers refer to the ability of older adults to maintain a positive sense of self and well-being despite losses associated with age as the *invulnerable self*. They suggest that older adults can maintain a high level of health, well-being, and life satisfaction despite changes in roles, relationships, and physical health. Lemme (1999) discussed some defenses used to protect the self, or how a person might maintain a positive sense of self. These include:

- Controlling information about our pasts through repression and selective recall
- Giving more weight to what we think about ourselves
- Not applying negative stereotypes to ourselves
- Interacting selectively in situations and with people who support our sense of self
- Identifying ourselves with a particular role, even though we no longer assume that role
- Discounting the importance of areas we are not good in
- Taking more credit for successes than failures
- Organizing our concepts of self so that the central core elements are positive attributes

Despite the fact that people with AD are faced with many losses associated with the disease, at times they can also maintain a positive sense of self. Although this adaptation often may not be deliberate or intentional, especially later in the disease, it can take place. At the same time, caregivers can function as facilitators of the process of adaptation for people with AD by creating supportive environments and interactions.

The Possible or Ideal Self

Some researchers discuss the notion of the ideal self or possible self—the self we are working toward or can imagine ourselves becoming. These potential selves can serve as important motivating forces for the individual. People create possible selves by projecting themselves into the future and thinking about what they would like to become, what they could become, and what they are afraid of becoming. Influences differ with age, as do the standards in which people use to judge themselves. Schaie and Willis (1996) discussed how Ryff identified six aspects of well-being: self-acceptance, positive relationships with others, autonomy, environmental mastery, purpose in life, and personal growth. The presence of possible selves in the self-report of middle-aged and older adults is seen as one of the salient predictors of successful aging. It is important to keep in mind that as individuals deal with change and loss associated with change, the possible or ideal self can be a motivating factor. This part of self may be the most difficult to uncover in people with AD or for the individual to formulate and communicate, especially later in the disease process. However, a person with AD may have shared this part of self with loved ones at some point throughout his or her life. Because of these unique circumstances, care environments and the interactions within them must become the support and motivation as people with AD are faced with loss and change.

Closing

Maintaining the self begins with an understanding of the self, its multidimensional nature and its formation in childhood and continued development throughout life. In understanding the self, the role and importance of others in the creation and validation of the self becomes clear. Research studies add another dimension and show us how this complex concept has been measured both quantitatively and qualitatively. Finally, we see the resiliency of the aging self and how it evolves and adapts with experience and situations. A background and knowledge of the self is important within the context of caring for individuals with Alzheimer's disease. This chapter serves as the foundation of learning toward creating a care community that recognizes the complexities and simplicities of the self. It is essential to apply what is known about the self to provide care that is truly person-centered. The next two chapters continue the discussion on the self. Chapter three describes how AD affects all aspects of a person, including identity, and Chapter Four reports findings from a research study shaped by existing theories of the self.

SELF-Reflection

EXAMINING WHAT SELF MEANS TO YOU

Think about what the self means to you. What has been significant in its development? How has it changed over time, and how do/did you incorporate those changes into your daily life? What *new* aspects of your self have been added in adulthood? What do you think your ideal or possible self might be?

Also, consider the multidimensional aspects of the self as described in Chapter Two. Think about the six domains—physical, social, emotional, intellectual, spiritual, and vocational. How do you identify yourself in each area, and how do you present each part of your self to others? Think about the types of activities, interactions, and environments you rely on to be successful in maintaining each different aspect of your self. Finally, think about what it would be like if you were no longer able to experience one or more parts of your self.

CHAPTER THREE

OVERVIEW OF ALZHEIMER'S DISEASE

I'm not living with Alzheimer's; Alzheimer's is living with me.

An adult day center participant with Alzheimer's disease

An estimated 5 million Americans have Alzheimer's disease (AD) (Alzheimer's Association, 2007). Additionally, one in ten people has a family member with AD, and one in three knows someone with AD (Alzheimer's Association, 2004). These statistics are staggering, and unless a cure or prevention is found, it is estimated that 11 million to 16 million Americans will have AD by 2050 (Alzheimer's Association, 2007).

This chapter includes a variety of information related to Alzheimer's disease. Some of the information you may have heard before, and other material may be new to you. At the same time, there are some additional thoughts on new ways of looking at the disease and on emerging thinking. This chapter provides general information on Alzheimer's disease and care, all in one place.

Dementia and Alzheimer's Disease

Alzheimer's disease is the most common cause of dementia. It is a progressive, degenerative disease of the brain that destroys brain cells, resulting in impairment of cognitive function. The symptoms associated with AD include memory loss, language and function impairment, and behavioral disturbances. Most conditions associated with dementia gradually destroy brain cells over time and lead to progressive decline in cognitive function. The rate of progression of dementia varies from person to person. The time from onset until death ranges from 3 to 20 years, with the average duration being 8 years (Alzheimer's Association, 2004).

Besides AD, another common form of dementia is vascular dementia, which results from reduced blood flow to the brain's nerve cells. Alzheimer's disease and vascular dementia can occur together and the condition is called *mixed dementia*. Other causes of dementia include Parkinson's disease, Creutzfeldt-Jakob disease, frontotemporal dementia, and dementia with Lewy bodies.

Warning Signs of Alzheimer's Disease

Memory changes associated with normal aging are different from symptoms of Alzheimer's disease. The Alzheimer's Association has developed a list of common symptoms to help people recognize that difference. Although this list can help to recognize symptoms, it is critical that concerned individuals be seen by a knowledgeable physician.

Ten Warning Signs of Alzheimer's

1. *Memory loss.* Forgetting names or appointments from time to time is normal, but forgetting recently learned information and forgetting more often and not being able to recall the information later is concerning.

2. *Difficulty performing familiar tasks.* Occasionally forgetting why you came into a room is normal, but finding it hard to plan and complete everyday tasks, such as preparing a meal or placing a call, is problematic.

3. *Problems with language.* Having trouble finding the right word sometimes is normal, but forgetting simple words or substituting with unusual words is problematic.

4. *Disorientation to time and place.* Not remembering the day of the week or where you were going is normal, but becoming lost in your own neighborhood is a reason for concern.

5. *Poor or decreased judgment.* Making a questionable decision occasionally is normal, but showing poor judgment in dressing and financial matters is concerning.

6. *Problems with abstract thinking.* Having difficulty balancing a checkbook is normal, but having trouble performing complex cognitive tasks, such as forgetting what numbers are for, is problematic.

7. *Misplacing things.* Not being able to find your keys is normal, but finding them in an unusual place, such as the freezer, is concerning.

8. *Changes in mood and behavior.* Feeling sad or moody from time to time is normal, but rapid mood swings for no apparent reason is something to be concerned about.

9. *Changes in personality.* As people age, personalities change; however, dramatic changes in personality, including suspiciousness or confusion, are a reason for concern.

10. *Loss of initiative.* Sometimes feeling weary of doing certain things is normal, but being passive for hours and not wanting to take part in usual activities is concerning.

Causes of Alzheimer's Disease

The neurological changes associated with AD include neocortical atrophy, neuron and synapse loss, and the presence of plaques and tangles (Salmon & Bondi, 1997). Many scientists believe that the damage in the brain begins years before any symptoms appear. AD is often attributed to plaques and tangles, which are clusters of proteins that accumulate in the brain and are considered to be directly observable hallmarks of AD (NIA, 2003). These plaques and tangles are either the cause of nerve cell death in the brain or the by-products of cell death. Researchers have not yet confirmed which is the case. Microscopic views of the Alzheimer's brain have revealed loss of nerve cells in certain brain regions, such as the hippocampus, a center for memory, and the cerebral cortex, which is involved in reasoning, memory, language, and other thought processes (St. George-Hyslop, 2000). As different areas of the brain become affected, additional cognitive abilities become impaired in addition to memory.

Diagnosis of Alzheimer's Disease

There is no single test to detect Alzheimer's disease. A diagnosis is based on a thorough evaluation of symptoms and an assessment of health. A knowledgeable neurologist or neuropsychologist conducts a variety of tests to assess memory and thinking skills and discusses changes in memory and behavior observed by family members. The neurologist or physician also conducts a thorough physical examination, reviews medical history, and orders a variety of laboratory tests that may include blood and urine samples or brain imaging scans (Alzheimer's Association, 2002). The physician may ask a family member or close friend about any noticeable change in the individual's memory, thinking skills, or behavior.

A skilled physician can diagnose Alzheimer's disease with 90% accuracy (Alzheimer's Association, 2006). Most diagnostic uncertainty comes from occasional difficulty distinguishing Alzheimer's disease from a related disorder. Diagnosis is very important to determine whether symptoms may be due to a condition other than dementia, such as depression, medication side effects, certain thyroid conditions, excess use of alcohol, and nutritional imbalances, which are all potentially treatable disorders that may sometimes impair memory or other cognitive functions (Alzheimer's Association, 2006). Even if the diagnosis is dementia, timely identification may allow individuals to take an active role in treatment decisions and in planning for the future.

Stages and Progression of Alzheimer's Disease

Several experts have developed a framework of stages to describe the progression of AD, documenting patterns of symptom development that generally correspond to the progressive degeneration of nerve cells. Although the stages can provide an understanding of how the disease may unfold, the progression of AD is very individual and can vary greatly from one person to another. If used inappropriately, therefore, stages can simply provide a framework for labeling people with the disease and may impose expectations about a person that limit or inhibit his or her contributions and abilities. From my experience, the most helpful and least restricting approach to disease stages is one that broadly recognizes early, middle, and late stages.

An often-used stage model developed by Dr. Barry Reisberg is outlined in the appendix to this chapter (see p. 53) (Alzheimer's Association, 2006). Alongside Reisberg's characterizations of loss and decline associated with each stage, an alternate description of strengths and abilities has been added. Although not perfect, the alternate descriptions can help us to think about how a more well-rounded representation can be helpful in individualized care. This alternate type of *staging* based on ability can be more helpful for care providers and family members as they develop care approaches that help maintain the self.

It is often believed that stages are needed to identify a predictable disease course and associated treatments. Stages typically focus on loss and decline, however, and not only illustrate a downward progression, but also tend to limit the uniqueness of the individual. They are restrictive in nature and often portray a solely dismal picture for families and professionals that is often untrue for this very individual disease. Sometimes, families will anticipate certain impairments and prematurely assign them to the individual, or they will refer to a *normal* behavior or action as a characteristic or symptom of a stage. Families and professionals are often heard referring to individuals as being *in stage 4*. This restrictive approach is not extremely helpful for care providers who are interested in strengths-based or person-centered care, nor for interactions that support or maintain the self. Sabat (2002) stated that all care providers must begin by recognizing that the many aspects of the cognitive life of people with dementia survive into the moderate to severe stages of the disease. These cognitive abilities include (but are not limited to) the ability to behave on the basis of the meaning of situations, to experience a range of emotions, to experience and seek to avoid embarrassment, to feel pride and seek to maintain self-respect, to feel concern for others, to communicate effectively with assistance from others, and to display at least implicit short-term and long-term memory.

Treatments for Alzheimer's Disease

There is no cure for AD. However, some treatments are available to slow the progression (or loss of nerve cells) and others to alleviate associated behaviors. There are even some treatments in development that may modify the disease progression. Some experts believe that these medications may also delay the need for nursing home care. In addition, there are many effective alternative and nonpharmacological treatments.

The U.S. Food and Drug Administration (FDA) has approved two drug classes—cholinesterase inhibitors and memantine—to treat cognitive symptoms of AD. Cholinesterase inhibitors are designed to prevent the breakdown of acetylcholine, a chemical messenger in the brain. It is said that approximately half of the individuals who take cholinesterase inhibitors initially experience a modest improvement in cognitive function (Alzheimer's Association, 2006).

The other FDA-approved drug class, memantine, is an N-methyl-D-aspartate (NMDA) receptor antagonist and works by regulating the activity of glutamate, one of the brain's specialized messenger chemicals used in information processing, storage, and retrieval. Glutamate triggers NMDA receptors to allow an appropriate amount of calcium to flow into a nerve cell, creating the chemical environment required for information storage (Alzheimer's Association, 2006). Excess glutamate overstimulates NMDA receptors, allowing too much calcium into the nerve cells and causing death of cells. Memantine may actually protect cells against excess glutamate by partially blocking NMDA receptors (Alzheimer's Association, 2006).

Another often-prescribed treatment for AD is vitamin E supplements. Some researchers believe that oxidative stress may play a role in Alzheimer's disease, and that a type of oxygen in the brain called free radicals can damage cells. Vitamin E supplements may actually defend against this type of damage. Most people can take vitamin E without side effects; however, the addition of or change in any medication should be discussed with a physician.

In addition to treatments for cognitive symptoms of AD, there are also treatments for behavioral and psychiatric symptoms that may occur with the disease. As the brain changes, some individuals experience symptoms such as anxiety and hallucinations. Many individuals, their families, and care providers find these types of symptoms to be the most challenging. Of course, a thorough medical assessment is necessary to decide on the most effective treatment and to determine potential underlying causes. Many times, non-drug interventions can be the most effective and appropriate. Deciding on treatments requires a careful and honest look at triggers and behaviors in the environment and in interactions with others.

Several alternative treatments have been identified for AD. Claims about safety and effectiveness of these herbal remedies and dietary supplements are based on a small body of scientific research. Since the rigor of FDA approval is not required for these treatments, it is important to use caution when considering them.

Finally, there are other nonpharmacological treatments that have been shown to be effective. What is classified as a nonpharmacological treatment, however, can vary greatly from source to source. Several examples include cognitive training, reminiscence, validation, creative arts therapy, psychotherapy, behavioral approaches, sensory interventions, physical exercise, and caregiver intervention. These types of approaches can improve cognitive functioning and optimize remaining abilities, decrease disruptive behaviors, and reduce distress, among other benefits. These types of treatment options are often overlooked, but may be very effective.

Types of Care Environments

Nearly 70% of people with AD are cared for in their homes and more often by spouses or adult children (Alzheimer's Association, 2007). A variety of home- and community-based care services are available to support individuals and their families in their homes. Services such as delivered meals, home modification, transportation, and homemaker services can provide assistance with daily needs. In addition, personal care and home health services can help with daily care needs. Adult day centers can provide a structured environment for individuals with AD while family members receive some time away from their care duties to accomplish other tasks, take part in other activities, or simply relax a bit. There are even respite camps and extended stay programs within some residential facilities for families needing a long break or for vacation needs.

Residential care is widely available for individuals who may need more care or a more structured/supportive care environment. Assisted living or group-type homes are an option for those who are mostly independent but who may need some assistance with tasks, such as house cleaning and daily reminders. As someone requires more care, a nursing home or long-term care facility can be the most appropriate care environment to meet his or her daily needs. Some facilities have separate floors or special care units that are specifically designed to meet the needs of individuals with AD and that have staff who are knowledgeable in caring for people with the disease. Today, there are even entire care facilities or campuses that have been designed specifically for individuals with AD.

Of course, care options vary from state to state, and the type of care can also vary from facility to facility. In any case, it is important that individuals with AD are in a care environment that specifically meets their unique needs and that they have care providers around them who are knowledgeable in Alzheimer's care.

Models of Alzheimer's Care

The traditional medical model of care is increasingly being seen as inappropriate for people with dementia. The medical model of dementia care, sometimes called the illness model, places emphasis on abnormalities in the structure and function of body organs that lead to disease. The disease, or problem, is the primary focus. Symptoms are seen as a direct result of the impairments that are inside the individual's body tissue, and it is assumed that these symptoms are attributed to the dysfunction of the body parts. At the same time, and as mentioned earlier, there is a continuous effort to outline stages of disease progression. It is often believed that stages are needed to identify a predictable disease course and associated treatments. The medical model of care does not take into consideration the uniqueness of dementia, the fact that symptoms often result from factors outside of the body, and that the disease progression varies from individual to individual.

In addition, the words used in the medical model are often impersonal and at times even military-like. Health care providers discuss wars to be won and diseases to be conquered and defeated. Often, discussions include phrases such as *administering a battery of tests*, *identifying the enemies*, and *developing a plan of attack*. There is usually a chief of staff, a head nurse on duty, and other charge nurses—all contributing to a perception of hierarchy, rigidity, and coldness.

Other models of care—such as social, psychosocial, or person-centered care, to name a few—are seen as more appropriate models for people with dementia. The philosophy of these types of care models are centered around the person, based on strengths and abilities, focused on collaboration and relationships, and flexible in nature. Language is typically more holistic, humanistic, and supportive in nature, focusing on partnership and solutions.

General descriptions of these types of models are outlined in Chapter One, and specific approaches within the models will be discussed in more detail in Sections II and III.

Emerging Thinking in Alzheimer's Care

The frame of thinking in the early 21st century among dementia care experts is moving beyond traditional models of and approaches to care in an effort to become more holistic and person-focused in nature. There is a general consensus that there is more to the disease than loss and decline, and that people can continue to lead productive and meaningful lives. There is a shared belief that care must be individualized and based on needs, interests, strengths, and abilities, and that relationships are key to the success. Pioneers such as Tom Kitwood and Steven Sabat have provided a philosophical and practical foundation that continues to be built upon by experts around the world. Chapter One already introduced some of these concepts, and the chapters that follow will highlight more work of these experts and build upon their concepts to further describe good care that supports the person.

Where to Go for Help

The Alzheimer's Association is the largest voluntary health organization dedicated to dementia research, care, and support. Local chapters throughout the country provide core services to families and professionals, including information and referral, support groups, care consultation, education, and safety services. In addition, there are many print and Internet resources as well as local aging organizations that may be helpful.

Closing

A solid understanding of Alzheimer's disease is key to providing good care and starts us on the journey of individualized care that supports the self. Traditional information and resources can provide us with general information, however new ways of thinking and organizing care can lend themselves to new perspectives and approaches to care. With all of the losses associated with AD, it is not surprising that professionals and family caregivers often assume a loss of identity. However, research and enlightened care practices have demonstrated that positive results can be seen when a person's identity or self is supported throughout the course of the disease, including improvements in functional ability, positive mood, food intake, and even physical health. The chapter that follows discusses research I conducted measuring the persistence of self in individuals with AD and reveals why the support of selfhood continues to be important throughout the course of the disease.

SELF-Reflection

DE-MEDICALIZING YOUR APPROACH TO CARE

Think about the care that is provided in your community. Is it based on the traditional medical model, is it psychosocial or person-centered, or is it somewhere in between? Consider the following general areas in relation to your care community. Talk with other staff as well as with families and try to capture your current ways of operating in these areas. Examine how medicalized the descriptions are or are not. Discuss together with other staff what can be done to become less medical in each area.

- Philosophical focus
- Words used
- Organizational structure
- Staff actions and approaches to care
- Involvement of person with dementia
- Environmental support

SELF-Reflection

EXAMINING MYTHS ABOUT ALZHEIMER'S DISEASE

Think about the following typical statements regarding Alzheimer's disease. For each, indicate whether the statement is true or false.

1. Memory loss is part of normal aging.

2. Aluminum causes Alzheimer's disease.

3. You can prevent Alzheimer's disease.

4. Alzheimer's disease is strictly a mental illness.

5. There are no treatments available for Alzheimer's disease.

6. The person with Alzheimer's disease does not understand what is going on around him or her.

7. All people with Alzheimer's disease eventually become violent and aggressive.

8. People with Alzheimer's disease eventually become completely helpless and cannot do anything for themselves.

9. Only families can provide good care for the person with Alzheimer's disease.

10. There is a cure for Alzheimer's disease.

All answers are false.

The Enduring Self in People with Alzheimer's. © 2008 by Health Professions Press.

APPENDIX: Stages of Alzheimer's disease—an alternative perspective

Loss/Decline	Strengths/Abilities

Stage 1: No impairment
Normal function

• Unimpaired individuals experience no memory problems and none are evident to a health care professional during a medical interview.	• Fully-functioning person

Stage 2: Very mild cognitive decline
May be normal age-related changes or earliest signs of Alzheimer's disease

• Individuals may feel as if they have memory lapses, especially in forgetting familiar words or names or the location of keys, eyeglasses, or other everyday objects. But these problems are not evident during a medical examination or apparent to friends, family, or co-workers.	• Fully functioning person who may forget something from time to time.

Stage 3: Mild cognitive decline
Early-stage Alzheimer's can be diagnosed in some, but not all, individuals with these symptoms.

Friends, family, or co-workers begin to notice deficiencies. Problems with memory or concentration may be measurable in clinical testing or discernible during a detailed medical interview. Common difficulties include:	A person remains able to:
• Word- or name-finding problems noticeable to family or close associates	• Engage in conversations with others although may need support with some words
• Decreased ability to remember names when introduced to new people • Performance issues in social or work settings noticeable to family, friends, or co-workers	• Meet new people and socialize although may not be able to refer to them by name all the time
• Reading a passage and retaining little material	• Enjoy reading short passages and stories
• Losing or misplacing a valuable object	• Locate misplaced items with help
• Decline in ability to plan or organize	• Plan uncomplicated tasks and activities or more complicated tasks with support and assistance

Appendix (Continued)

Loss/Decline	Strengths/Abilities

Stage 4: Moderate cognitive decline
Mild or early-stage Alzheimer's disease

Loss/Decline	Strengths/Abilities
At this stage, a careful medical interview detects clear-cut deficiencies in the following areas:	A person continues to be able to:
• Decreased knowledge of recent occasions or current events	• Talk about the past in great detail
• Impaired ability to perform challenging mental arithmetic—for example, to count backward from 100 by 7s	• Perform basic arithmetic
• Decreased capacity to perform complex tasks, such as marketing, planning dinner for guests, or paying bills and managing finances	• Perform noncomplex tasks or more complex tasks with assistance
• Reduced memory of personal history	• Have memory of personal history with reminders or cues
• The affected individual may seem subdued and withdrawn, especially in socially or mentally challenging situations	• Engage in social and mentally challenging situations when included appropriately or in a simplified manner

Stage 5: Moderately severe cognitive decline
Moderate or mid-stage Alzheimer's disease

Loss/Decline	Strengths/Abilities
Major gaps in memory and deficits in cognitive function emerge. Some assistance with day-to-day activities becomes essential. At this stage, individuals may:	At this stage, individuals can:
• Be unable during a medical interview to recall such important details as their current address, their telephone number, or the name of the college or high school from which they graduated	• Convey feelings
• Become confused about where they are or about the date, day of the week, or season	• Be in and enjoy the moment
• Have trouble with less challenging mental arithmetic; for example, counting backward from 40 by 4s or from 20 by 2s	• Perform simple mental arithmetic

Appendix (Continued)

Loss/Decline	Strengths/Abilities
• Need help choosing proper clothing for the season or the occasion	• Select clothing with limited choices
• Retain substantial knowledge about themselves and know their own name and the names of their spouse or children	• Have knowledge about themselves and know names of spouse and children
• Require no assistance with eating or using the toilet	• Eat and use bathroom independently

Stage 6: Severe cognitive decline
Moderately severe or mid-stage Alzheimer's disease

Memory difficulties continue to worsen, significant personality changes may emerge, and affected individuals need extensive help with customary daily activities. At this stage, individuals may:	At this stage, individuals can:
• Lose most awareness of recent experiences and events, as well as of their surroundings	• Talk about past experiences in some detail
• Recollect their personal history imperfectly, although they generally recall their own name	• Know their name and recall personal history with cues
• Occasionally forget the name of their spouse or primary caregiver but generally can distinguish familiar from unfamiliar faces	• Recognize familiar faces and individuals
• Need help getting dressed properly; without supervision, may make such errors as putting pajamas over daytime clothes or shoes on wrong feet	• Dress self with limited choices and support or assistance
• Experience disruption of their normal sleep/waking cycle	• Enjoy an afternoon nap or early morning sunrise
• Need help with handling details of toileting (flushing toilet, wiping and disposing of tissue properly)	• Use the bathroom with cues and support/assistance
• Have increasing episodes of urinary or fecal incontinence	• Use toilet and be successful with reminders

Appendix (Continued)

Loss/Decline	Strengths/Abilities
• Experience significant personality changes and behavioral symptoms, including suspiciousness and delusions (for example, believing that their caregiver is an impostor); hallucinations (seeing or hearing things that are not really there); or compulsive, repetitive behaviors such as hand-wringing or tissue shredding	• Perform or assist with tasks that are repetitive in nature
• Tend to wander and become lost	• Move around and take walks with supervision

Stage 7: Very severe cognitive decline
Severe or late-stage Alzheimer's disease

This is the final stage of the disease when individuals lose the ability to respond to their environment, the ability to speak, and, ultimately, the ability to control movement. At this stage, individuals:	At this stage, individuals can:
• Frequently lose their capacity for recognizable speech, although words or phrases may occasionally be uttered	• Use simple words or phrases, and is often able to respond nonverbally or with groans
• Need help with eating and toileting and there is general incontinence of urine	• Eat with assistance and use the bathroom with assistance
• Lose the ability to walk without assistance, then the ability to sit without support, the ability to smile, and the ability to hold their head up; reflexes become abnormal and muscles grow rigid; swallowing is impaired.	• Walk with help and sit with support • Enjoy tastes of certain flavors

CHAPTER FOUR

EVIDENCE OF THE SELF IN ALZHEIMER'S DISEASE

The self is more than memory. It is forged on a continuum of memory and creativity that exists in a social context.

Anne Basting (2003)

Many studies have been conducted on the self and Alzheimer's disease (AD). These are summarized in this chapter along with research that I have conducted regarding the persistence of self in individuals with AD, as shown through visual self-recognition and use of language. For those who are interested, my study's formal procedures and results are presented in an appendix at the end of the book. This chapter provides a discussion of the study results in a context that, taken together with the preceding chapters, provides the foundation for the Alzheimer's care practices that are described in the chapters that follow.

What We Know

Information on the diagnosis, assessment, and progression of AD is abundant and many resources are available for care providers and professionals to assist them in providing care. However, the way in which the symptoms and changes related to AD impact the self has only begun to be explored in the research and care communities. Also, the instruments commonly used to assess self are not appropriate for the Alzheimer's population, such as use of mirrors and self-report measures, and can present many challenges. As a result, many of the studies that have explored self in individuals with AD have

The author would like to acknowledge Dr. David Mitchell for his contributions to this project and chapter.

been unsuccessful in applying common measurement techniques or have been qualitative or descriptive in nature because of the challenges in measuring such a concept.

Typical Portrayals of Alzheimer's Disease

Negative terms are commonly used to characterize individuals with AD and their experience with the disease. Words such as *victim, sufferer,* and *shell* are often used to describe the person with the disease, and the experience of the disease is often described as a *living death, never-ending funeral,* or *private hell of devastation and destruction* (Lushin, 1990). Herskovits (1995) stated that the typical portrayals of Alzheimer's and their widespread acceptance and popularization have significant consequences, specifically to the self. A medicalized approach to caring for and the stigmatization and objectification of individuals with AD, as well as thinking of the experience of Alzheimer's as the *loss* or *death* of self, are examples of some of the more common negative aspects of AD (Herskovits, 1995). The overwhelming and dominant negative effect of the current portrayals of AD is the dehumanization and debasement of self (Herskovits, 1995). For instance, Robertson (1991) stated, "Alzheimer's disease represents the loss of all those qualities by which we have come to define our humanness" (p. 143). Other researchers have described the disease as the unbecoming of self (Fontana & Smith, 1989) and, more commonly, as the loss of self (Cohen & Eisdorfer, 1986). However, the portrayal of Alzheimer's as a loss of self is not an accurate one, as the data discussed in this chapter will show, and the implications of such negative characterizations can be detrimental to the care and treatment of individuals with the disease.

Lyman (1989) described the current view of dementia as an example of the *medicalization of deviance,* which she defines as treating the person and social troubles as medical problems. Lyman argued that the medical model includes many disease categories that limit the self-identity of the person with dementia and suggested a shift in how AD is perceived to include social factors and the recognition of the individual. Harrison (1993) stated that a medical focus, which looks only at problems, should also assess the individual's remaining strengths, positive functions, and characteristics. Harrison suggested that we examine what makes a person the same person over time, and reinforced the notion that personhood is more than just cognitive abilities and includes many additional facets and contexts. Kitwood (1988) also discussed the importance of maintaining personhood and suggested that as the individual is continually invalidated and objectified, he or she loses more and more of the vital contact with others that personhood depends upon.

Supporting the whole self is a fundamental component of maintaining personhood. A medical approach to caring for someone with dementia fails to appreciate the disease from the person's point of view and fails to support the complete and lifelong self (Morris, 1996).

Visual Self-Recognition Techniques

Following the example of successful studies with young children, several researchers have studied the concept of self in people with dementia using mirror-recognition techniques (Biringer & Anderson, 1992; Grewal, 1994). Biringer and Anderson (1992) examined self-recognition in individuals with AD using both mirror and video techniques. Using the Global Deterioration Scale as an index, they found that all participants with moderate dementia showed self-recognition in the mirror, whereas 25% of participants with moderately severe dementia did not recognize themselves. At the same time, only 7 out of 29 participants in both groups together showed signs of self-recognition on video.

In a related study, Grewal (1994) studied self-recognition in people with dementia using body part naming and mirror recognition. Of the 39 individuals who were tested, 20 were diagnosed with moderate dementia and 19 with severe dementia. The findings suggested that individuals with moderate dementia are still capable of self-recognition; however, as the disease progresses and the dementia becomes more severe, the ability no longer exists. In another study on self-recognition and people with dementia, Gil et al. (2001) found that the least disturbed aspects of self-consciousness were awareness of identity and of mental representation of the body. The most disturbed aspects were awareness of cognitive deficiencies, moral judgments, and prospective memory or remembering to do something.

The use of mirrors in visual self-recognition studies is commonplace. However, it is not uncommon for individuals with dementia to experience difficulties with their images in the mirror. Mirrors may be confusing and misinterpreted as a second person in the room (Petersen, 2002). In several studies, individuals with AD have demonstrated the *mirror sign*, or the inability to recognize the reflection of oneself in a mirror (Phillips, Howard & David, 1996). Other studies have shown a person's inability to recognize his or her image as that of his or her own, misidentification of his or her image as someone else's, and even agitated behavior resulting from mirror–self misperception (Forstl et al., 1994; Mendez et al., 1992; Molchan et al., 1990). These studies demonstrate that testing self-recognition with mirrors might present some challenges for individuals with AD.

Narrative Techniques

Research using narrative techniques to study self in AD has gleaned somewhat different findings than the self-recognition studies (Sabat, 2002; Sabat & Collins, 1999; Sabat & Harre, 1992; Tappen et al., 1999). Sabat and Harre (1992) examined the loss of self in AD in relation to a social constructionist view of the nature of self, stating, "Selfhood is publicly manifested in various discursive practices, such as telling autobiographical stories, taking on the responsibility of one's actions, expressing doubt, declaring interest in care, decrying the lack of fairness in a situation, and so on" (p. 445). Through case studies of three individuals, they suggested that Self1, the self of personal identity, persists far into the end stage of the disease. Self2, the multiple personae presented in public and with the help of others, can be lost, but only indirectly as a result of how others treat and view the person with AD. Sabat and Harre suggested that losses in aspects of selfhood might be traced to dysfunctional social interactions rather than to the neuropathology of the disease. In addition, they proposed that it is not intact memory that constitutes one's self or one's personal identity in the sense of self, and that the use of first-person pronouns can count for indicators of personhood (Sabat & Harre, 1992).

Sabat and Collins (1999) expanded upon these findings with an individual case study and found intact social and cognitive abilities as well as intact manifestations of selfhood as viewed from a social constructivist point of view. They identified three ways in which a person's selfhood can be expressed: Self1, or the personal identity, which is manifested in the use of personal pronouns; Self2, or one's attributes (past and present), beliefs, and beliefs about attributes; and Self3, or the public persona that is manifested with the help of others in our social world (Sabat & Collins, 1999). Despite significant impairments in the cognitive abilities of the case study participant, the researchers found indications of self within all three expressions of selfhood.

Sabat (2002) expanded even further upon this model by explaining Self1, Self2, and Self3 in more detail. Self1, self of personal identity, refers to the continuity of one's singular and unique point of view. It is not dependent on one's personal history or ability to account recent history since it pertains more to ownership. Self2, self of mental and physical attributes, refers to how a person describes himself or herself, including attitudes, feelings, and beliefs. Self3, socially presented selves or personae, refers to how we present Self2 to others. This self is dependent on others to support and maintain it. In brief, Self1 is the person's sense of continuity across time, Self2 links the person's present and past experiences, and Self3 is his or her social display of self (Bender, 2003).

Sabat (2002) also added a new component to Self2 that included deficits related to the neuropathology of the disease. This revision addressed early findings that suggested a connection between self and the interaction or relationship with healthy others. He concluded that it is possible to observe intact self or selves in individuals with Alzheimer's disease through language (Sabat, 2002). Sabat and Harre (1992) summarized their findings as demonstrating an internally defined self (self) and externally defined self (persona). Herskovits (1995) drew similar conclusions, describing the nature of self as a combination of an internal personal identity and an intersubjective public and social project.

Several other researchers have examined the self as an internal personal identity through the measurement of pronoun use. Bender (2003) found 8 examples of I, me, mine, and ours per 100 words for people who were identified as *confused* by the Clifton Assessment Procedures for the Elderly (CAPE); 7 uses per 100 words for those who were *nonconfused*; and 6.5 uses for the control group. Bender and his colleagues found that the cognitively impaired individuals did not lose the concept of I and that they, in fact, used it significantly more often than the other groups. They concluded, "So it would appear that I-ness is resistant to cognitive losses and, to the extent that it measures or reflects Self1, Self1 appears to be the enduring feature of the person" (p. 247). Their theory is context-elicited and assumes variability across contexts and environments.

Small et al. (1998) also studied the internal and external self in people with dementia, expanding upon the findings of Sabat and Harre (1992). They found that 8 out of 17 individuals with severe cognitive impairment used first-person singular pronouns. In addition to verbal behaviors, Small et al. (1998) also examined nonverbal behaviors of individuals with dementia, and of their caregivers, and concluded that personal pronouns alone are not sufficient for determining the integrity of self and that other forms of language and nonverbal behavior are necessary to measure selfhood. In another study, Hubbard et al. (2002) examined nonverbal behavior in individuals with dementia and also concluded that certain nonverbal behaviors can be seen as interpretations of self. The nonverbal behaviors were found to be used to amplify meaning of verbal communication, to remain part of a communicative world, and to compensate for loss of verbal abilities. Specific nonverbal behaviors included facial expressions, postures, proximity, gestures, and physical contact with inanimate objects.

Tappen et al. (1999) also expanded upon the view proposed by Sabat and Harre (1992) and used conversational analysis to examine the persistence of a sense of self or personal identity in advanced AD. They found that respondents used the first-person pronouns frequently, freely, and coherently. These findings are similar to Sabat's in that they support a persistence of awareness of self during the middle and late stages of the disease. Kolanowski and Whall (1996) also presented evidence for the continuity of personality in dementia. They found that although there were systematic shifts in personality, individuals with dementia tend to maintain their former personality traits. As a whole, these findings lend support to the continued existence of self in individuals with AD.

New Research on the Persistence of Self in Individuals with Alzheimer's Disease

This study was designed to combine both visual self-recognition and narrative techniques. Based on the premise that the characterization of AD as *a loss of self* is not accurate, the study had two goals: (1) to analyze language for evidence of self references and (2) to examine visual self-recognition for evidence of the persistence of self in individuals with AD. Regarding language, it was hypothesized that in spite of declines in the frequency of pronoun and attribute use across levels of cognitive impairment (cf. Lyons et al., 1994), similarities should be evident in more subtle linguistic indications of self-knowledge. Evidence for self should be found if some of the cognitive and language deficits can be bypassed. Regarding visual measures, in light of the problems encountered with the use of mirrors, recent instant photographs were used instead. It was hypothesized that there should be no differences in visual self-recognition across levels of cognitive impairment (mild to moderate).

Overview

The study was conducted with 78 English-speaking older adults (ages 66 to 103), the majority of whom were Caucasian females with a high degree of education. They were divided into three groups: one with no impairment, a second with mild impairment, and a third with moderate impairment. For each group with cognitive impairments, half of the individuals resided in the community and attended an adult day center and half were in a residential facility. The participants were interviewed for approximately 15 minutes on average using questions developed to encourage discussion of the person's self in relation to the following attribute categories, which are based on Sabat and Collins (1999) and Sabat and Harre (1992):

- Physical traits
  - Lifelong
  - Disease-focused

- Personal characteristics and qualities
  - Lifelong
  - Disease-focused
- Familial
- Vocational or professional
- Educational
- Talents, hobbies, and interests
- Attitudes and beliefs
  - Lifelong
  - Disease-focused

The interviewer progressed from general and nonthreatening questions, such as "Tell me about yourself" and "How would you describe what you look like?," to more specific questions, such as "What is your philosophy of life?" and "What do you hope for and dream about?" If needed, a general probe of "Anything else?" or a targeted probe of "Can you tell me more about ____?" was used.

For the self-recognition portion of the study, each participant's photograph was taken with an instant camera. In the individual test, each participant was shown his or her own picture approximately 3 minutes after it was taken and was asked, "Can you tell me who the person is in this photograph?" In the group test, each participant was shown a group of five photographs. One was the participant's own picture taken earlier in the visit and the other four were of strangers of the same gender and similar age. The participant was asked, "Can you tell me which of these photographs is you?" The group test came at the end of the spoken interview.

Specific details regarding the research method and results of the study can be found in the appendix.

Discussion of Study Findings

The results of the study demonstrate a persistence of self across three levels of cognitive impairment. Personhood is more than just cognitive abilities (Harrison, 1993). Both the language and visual recognition data gleaned from the study support this claim. Too much emphasis has been placed on the role of memory in determining and demonstrating the persistence of self.

Language Use

Although overall word use declined as impairment increased, many pronouns and attributes were still prominent during the interviews, suggesting persistence of self in even moderate dementia. These results are consistent with other reports. Shenk et al. (2002) identified specific markers of social identity, including proper names and geographic locations, that link the past to the present. Their study found evidence for the social-identity self through the persistence of representations of personal and social identity, as shown by continued use of pronouns and attributes across increased levels of cognitive impairment.

In further support of the persistence of self, the rates of language use revealed that participants at each level of cognitive impairment produced similar numbers of pronouns and attributes per minute. Individuals with cognitive impairments talked less overall (i.e., fewer total references), but compared to their total language production they were still able to produce pronouns and attributes at rates very similar to those without impairments. This suggests that it is not a loss of self per se that is responsible for a lower frequency of language use, but more likely a decreased ability to initiate conversation. Effective communication may require greater and more appropriate support from others. Indeed, Small et al. (1998) cautioned against measuring the self solely by pronoun counts or other simple quantitative language indicators. As cognitive impairment progresses, language becomes increasingly impaired (NIA, 2003), as do the abilities to communicate effectively and to initiate conversation (Petersen, 2002). Froggatt (1988) described a distinction between the cognitive self, which may be affected by memory loss, and the feeling self, which may be less impaired but be hampered by the inability to verbalize.

The proportions of types of pronouns and attributes used were also similar across all three levels of cognitive impairment. There were no significant differences in the use of the pronouns *I*, *myself*, *my*, *implicit* ("brown hair"), or *plural* ("We have two children"). Consistent with findings described by Bender (2003), *I* was the most frequently used pronoun for all participants, regardless of impairment level. Proportionally, there were also no significant differences across impairment levels in the attribute categories analyzed in the study: physical traits–lifelong, physical traits–disease focused, personal characteristics–lifelong, personal characteristics–disease focused, familial, vocational, educational, and talents, hobbies, and interests.

In people with dementia, Cohen-Mansfield et al. (2000) found that family roles retained the most prominence in the present. In their study, familial and attitudes–lifelong were the most frequently referenced attribute categories across levels of cognitive impairment. The categories that persisted can provide important markers to enhance communication and maintain the self through interaction with others. Additionally, diseased-focused attributes were not used frequently by participants. This finding is consistent with the literature that asserts that the self is socially supported and maintained, as the interview guide was designed to support a multidimensional, lifelong self rather than a disease-focused self.

The majority of participants with cognitive impairments had difficulties finding words and showed facial signs of confusion. They often stated that they could not remember, talked around subjects, and lingered on previous questions or stories. A prosthetic or supportive environment that would allow individuals with cognitive impairments to communicate more successfully might yield more significant indicators of self.

Visual Indicators of Self

This study revealed only minor differences in visual self-recognition across levels of cognitive impairment in the individual and group test conditions. These results support the assertion that there is a persistence of self in cognitively impaired individuals. Since previous research had revealed difficulties with self-recognition using mirrors in people with dementia, the use of photographs seemed to be the most appropriate approach and may have allowed for successful self-recognition.

Lack of movement may have been the key variable in accounting for the success with photographs. As opposed to mirrors and videos, photographs offer a still image that perhaps facilitates focus, without distraction. On the other hand, Biringer and Anderson (1992) found that self-recognition ability in the later stages of AD persisted longer for mirrors than for videos. Unfortunately, no still photos were included in their study.

Although the majority of participants were successful in the individual and group conditions, three participants with moderate cognitive impairments did not self-recognize in the individual condition and made comments to that effect. And nine participants with mild or moderate cognitive impairments who did successfully self-recognize in the individual condition made comments that indicated that they did not recall that the photograph was just taken by the investigator approximately three minutes earlier. These participants showed signs of self-recognition or self-awareness in spite of recall difficulties (see the study results in the Appendix).

The group test condition might have been easier than the individual test condition, because participants were asked to make a choice among five same-gender and racially and ethnically different photographs. Alternatively, the task of picking oneself from within a group may not have seemed as odd as asking the participant in the individual condition to identify him- or herself in a single photograph. Although the individual test condition may have seemed *absurd* or *bizarre* to the nonimpaired participants, none offered any comments or incredulous looks, except for a couple of chuckles. Perhaps the individual condition was more akin to a mirror condition, albeit with a static image.

The mechanisms that mediate the sense of self and of self-recognition may be separate from those that mediate the recall of recent events or episodes. Using functional magnetic resonance imaging (fMRI), Johnson et al. (2002) investigated the neurological processes underlying self-reflection. Healthy participants responded to statements requiring knowledge of and reflection on their self, as characterized by their abilities, traits, and attitudes. Their fMRI data revealed that frontal temporal networks were activated during self-reflective thought. Although the participants did not have cognitive impairments, the findings may help explain why participants in our study were able to self-recognize while simultaneously being unable to remember their picture being taken only minutes earlier. Cortical activation is correlated with self-awareness and episodic memory in different areas of the brain (see also Craik et al., 1999). The hippocampus, which is essential for episodic memory, is impaired by AD, whereas self-awareness is mediated primarily by the frontal lobe, an area typically unaffected by the disease (Budson & Price, 2005; Salmon & Bondi, 1997; St. George-Hyslop, 2000). This might explain why participants could successfully self-recognize in spite of memory difficulties.

Qualitative Analyses

The content of what participants discussed was analyzed by themes. Several themes were similar across the three levels of cognitive impairment and are highlighted in the pages that follow to illustrate these similarities. These themes included statements regarding war, the Depression, women's roles, and the focus of hopes and dreams. Below are a few statements from each of the three groups.

War. Many participants discussed their involvement in war, or about the effects of war on their lives. Statements from participants with no cognitive impairments include the following:

> "Since I was overseas when he died [brother], I couldn't come back for his funeral. That still leaves a hole in my heart."

> "And then I got married, because World War II had started and everyone got married before the guys went away."

Statements from participants with mild cognitive impairments include the following:

"I was in the war, and a vicious one I didn't like. But, when you gotta' kill you don't like it. . . . I don't like to kill. Either I kill or go to court martial."

"I was married to my first love, we was together six months and he had to go to war and I never seen him again."

Statements from participants with moderate cognitive impairments include the following:

"My husband died in World War II. He was never found."

"I'm a retired military, so I've traveled a bit and I've been in a few wars, so it's good to get home to my family."

The Depression. Participants also discussed the effects of the Depression on their lives. Statements from participants with no cognitive impairment include the following:

"I grew up in the Depression, which was very, very hard. That is why none of us were able to go to college when we were younger. We all had to go to work immediately."

"My parents had a jewelry store, but they lost that during the Depression . . . so both my parents had to work then. It was tough times living in the Depression."

Statements from participants with mild cognitive impairments include the following:

"We didn't have very many dollars to throw around and we had had a comfortable way until I was at least through seventh grade, then I realized there had been something called the Depression and I'd begun to learn what it meant."

"I couldn't get a job right away as a secretary because it was the Depression. That was the worst time in the world."

Statements from participants with moderate cognitive impairments include the following:

"When school come around I was limited to the type of work I could do, especially during the Depression."

"I'm from the Depression you know. I did housework. I did menial types of jobs. I was content—did my jobs well and made it."

Women's roles. Many female participants discussed their expected roles as women. This discussion often included how they were not encouraged to do or be much, and how they wished they had done more. Statements from participants with no cognitive impairment include:

"When I was a little girl he [father] told me that the stork made a mistake and should have delivered a boy. He always made sort of derogatory remarks when someone's child turned out to be a girl—'well it was only a girl.'"

"My parents didn't encourage college for us girls."

"I started working on my Master's, but my husband got very upset because I would have more education than he had. This was another era, so I stopped that, which was dumb, but anyway."

"Later on, when I went to NYC, there was no jobs. The only job for women was a domestic job, so that's what I took."

Statements from participants with mild cognitive impairments include the following:

"Before I married, and that's the only time I worked professionally."

"The ladies had to take a certain amount of education, and you had to choose a choice. You could either choose music or art, but they didn't want them to do any math because that was like men."

"I had to take a commercial course. I love art and music and would have loved to have taken a different course, but my mother was a widow and so we had to take a course so we could get a job. So I took a commercial course—so I took typewriting and shorthand and bookkeeping. So that's what I did."

Statements from participants with moderate cognitive impairments include the following:

"I was always a secretary. Years ago, when you were a personal secretary that was a nice thing to be."

"I worked there for about a year but then Mama died and I had to go home and take care of the children."

"I had to drop out of school because I had children."

Hopes for family members. Many participants shared hopes about the health and well-being of their family members. Statements from participants with no cognitive impairments include:

"I hope I see my great-grandchildren grow up and that I get to enjoy them."

"I hope that Frank [partner] will be in my life as healthy as he can be for longer."

"Well, I hope that my two youngest boys find their ways. I hope that all my children will be happy and have successful lives."

Statements from participants with mild cognitive impairments include the following:

"I am very lucky to have had three children and they are all doing very well right now. I think that's a mother's hope, that she sees everything turn out the way she wants it."

"The two people in my life that are ill, I try to do things so something will drift toward them."

"I hope to see my grandchildren grow up."

Statements from participants with moderate cognitive impairments include the following:

"I hope, I wish my mother was still with me."

"I tell the grandchildren to be good in school. I tell them to keep them in school so they can have a better life. I hope the best for them."

"I hope that, now being selfish, thinking about my family. First fold, that my husband and I can get along a little bit longer. I also hope that I have put enough into my children so they have some sense and do the right thing."

The themes described above were evident across all three levels of cognitive impairment. In addition, the themes in the content of what participants discussed were similar across the three groups.

What the Study May Mean for Care

Perhaps AD can be understood differently. Characterizations such as *the loss of self* might be altered to represent the disease more accurately. Care providers and family members can be made aware that the self does persist in individuals with AD, but that it also requires their active support to be maintained. Interactions should focus on supporting the lifelong characteristics of the self and not the disease-focused self (based solely on symptoms and problems). Care environments can be designed to better recognize and support the lifelong self by gathering appropriate information and by structuring activities and interactions to support aspects of the remaining self. As one's self is supported and maintained, an individual with AD may have a less negative disease experience.

Closing

Research has shown us how the self is affected by dementia, and more specifically how the persistence of self can be measured and discussed. The new research discussed in this chapter illustrates how the self can be measured through visual self-recognition and language use. The self remains, however the ability to initiate and maintain it is impaired. We have begun to see how important other people are in creating environments and interactions that are reflective and supportive of a lifelong self, thus allowing it to persist in Alzheimer's care. The chapters that follow outline specific ways for caregivers to support and maintain the self.

SELF-Reflection

THINKING ABOUT THE PERSISTENCE OF SELF

This chapter outlined how the persistence of self was measured through visual self-recognition and through the language individuals used to talk about themselves. It also discussed a variety of other approaches to measuring self in the literature today.

Take some time to think about the persistence of self in individuals with dementia who you know. What are some indicators of self that you have seen? What are some indicators of self that you might not have noticed? Begin to think about how interactions and the environment can play roles in the persistence of self.

SECTION II

ESSENTIAL ELEMENTS
OF CARE THAT
SUPPORT SELFHOOD

CHAPTER FIVE

PHYSICAL AND SOCIAL ENVIRONMENTS THAT RECOGNIZE THE SELF

Home is when I'm with people I care about and who care about me.

Person with dementia

Environment is an important factor in good care and must be structured in ways that recognize and support the self. Some of those ways may be reflected in the physical environment; however, many of them are realized in social or cultural environments or in the interactions, relationships, and approaches that take place within the physical environment. This chapter outlines overarching themes to consider to be sure the environment in your community is supportive of individual identity and helps maintain selfhood.

Key Elements in Environmental Design for Dementia Care

There are many resources available that discuss environment and how to construct one that promotes good dementia care. There are various elements of the physical environment, as well as social interactions within the physical environment, that are important to consider in creating a supportive setting that recognizes the self.

Margaret Calkins has done a lot of writing and research in environmental design and dementia care. In *Key Elements of Dementia Care*, Calkins and Sloane (1997) described 10 goals of environmental design. Rather than discussing specific details of design in each area, the 10 goals are provided below as a framework for discussion about environmental design in relation to maintaining the self.

Maximize Awareness and Orientation

The amount and type of support needed to maintain awareness and orientation is very individual. Design elements within environments can help to maximize awareness and orientation without being overwhelming and confusing. A common option is a personalized room entry with biography boards. Room entries are clearly identified with boards featuring photographs of that person. Not only does this option assist with orientation and awareness, but it also can contribute to the maintenance of selfhood.

Ensure Safety and Security

Of course, people with dementia need to be in environments that are safe and secure. Supportive options rather than restrictive ones are most appropriate for maintaining selfhood. Creating a safe and secure environment can be reflected in the way we communicate, provide care, and interact with individuals.

Provide Privacy

Personal space is important to everyone, including people with dementia. They, too, need a place to be alone or with others in a private setting. Room dividers or positioning of furniture can be helpful for shared rooms, and small gathering rooms should be made available for private time and for visits with others.

Support Functional Abilities

Environments should be designed in ways that support functional abilities and that build on individual strengths. Support (physical, personal, emotional) and assistance should be available so that individuals can be successful in applying their functional abilities.

Adjust the Amount of Stimulation

Many behaviors that are seen as disruptive or harmful can be a result of too much stimulation and activity within an environment. To reduce these types of behaviors and to support the functional capabilities of individuals with AD, an environment must be designed in ways to reduce unnecessary noise and overstimulation.

Provide Positive Quality Stimulation

Certain stimulation is good and necessary, and an environment must be designed to support and encourage that type of stimulation. People with dementia should have opportunities within an environment to be stimulated appropriately and to be able to connect to things that are important and that can maintain their selfhood.

Provide Opportunities for Personal Control

Everyone needs to feel in control of his or her situation and environment. This can be overlooked in care settings in which all decisions often are made for the residents. Individuals should be provided opportunities to have a say in a variety of situations. This can be as simple as deciding what to wear, how to spend the day, or when to eat. It can also include how to decorate one's room or public spaces. Individuals may also be included in larger decisions or discussions about the community, in whichever ways make sense and are appropriate.

Facilitate Social Contact

As will be discussed in Chapter Six, social interactions with others help to maintain who we are, or our self. We all require some sort of social interaction, although how much and what type varies from person to person. We have the ability to initiate what form of social contact we want and when we want it. That ability to initiate often does not exist for people with dementia. Staff need to find ways to facilitate appropriate social interaction. Physical spaces and activities can be designed to encourage a range of social interactions.

Maintain Self-Identity

Maintaining self-identity is essential to preserving the self. Physical, social, and cultural environments must be designed to maintain self-identity. Living settings should allow for personalization throughout the community, not only in a resident's bedroom. Wherever possible, rooms should contain images and objects that are meaningful to the resident and that represent who he or she has been throughout his or her life and not only who he or she is now. The combination and interplay of both is essential for maintaining self-identity.

Adapt to Disease Continuum

Finally and most importantly, each environment and social interaction needs to be continually evaluated and adapted to address changes in functional ability, cognitive status, and communication as the disease progresses. At the same time, an environment must be able to meet the needs of the evolving self throughout the continuum of the disease.

In her book *Creating Successful Dementia Care Settings*, Calkins continued to develop a thematic approach to design. These themes are helpful in encouraging us to think about possibilities rather than prescribing specific details or actions. Calkins (2001) discussed the following three themes in environmental design for people with dementia: (1) enhance identity and sense of being at home; (2) support functional independence; and (3) minimize distress and behaviors that are disruptive to the self and to others.

Identity and a sense of being at home can be enhanced by including a resident's personal items inside and outside of his or her bedroom. Functional independence can be supported and encouraged through approaches to dressing, use of the bathroom, and eating. Finally, distress and behaviors that are disruptive to others can be minimized by creating settings within an environment where certain behaviors are acceptable or encouraged. These three design themes can be used to create good care environments for people with dementia as well as care environments that help to support the self.

Calkins (2002) also discussed the nursing home of the future and how the overall movement generally includes the following goals: (1) respecting the individualized needs and desires of each person; (2) honoring the life patterns and accomplishments of every person within the setting; (3) supporting opportunities for continued growth; (4) enabling continued productive contributions to the community; (5) encouraging meaningful connections with family and the community; and (6) fostering fun. These goals can also be useful in thinking about creating dementia care environments.

Other pioneers in environmental design and Alzheimer's care have developed design principles that could serve as guidelines in considering the needs of any specific community. In *Holding onto Home*, Cohen and Weisman (1991) described therapeutic goals in environmental design. Brawley (1997) stated that therapeutic goals are intended to provide direction in creating appropriate and supportive environments. They can be used as guidelines in defining the relationships and interactions between individuals with dementia and their environments. They can also provide direction for design decisions, program development, and overall policy. Cohen and Weisman (1991) identified the following therapeutic goals:

1. Ensure safety and security.

2. Support functional ability through meaningful activity.

3. Maximize awareness and orientation.

4. Provide opportunities for stimulation and change.

5. Maximize autonomy and control.

6. Adapt to changing needs.

7. Establish links to the healthy and familiar.

8. Provide opportunities for socialization.

9. Protect the need for privacy.

10. Encourage family involvement (suggested as an addition by Brawley, 1997).

These goals can be used as guidelines as you create and re-create supportive environments for people with dementia.

Cohen and Weisman (1991) also discussed some general attributes of the environment that should influence the overall design of spaces. These design principles include noninstitutional appearance and characteristics, elimination of environmental barriers, incorporation of things from the past, and sensory stimulation without stress. Applying one or each of these principles can encourage the development of specific strategies to create environments and interactions within them that support person-centered care and the self.

When thinking about the environment, it is useful to consider both public and private spaces. As mentioned earlier, it is important to find ways to support the self beyond a resident's bedroom. Think about how public spaces such as dining rooms, living rooms, and hallways can include personal items of the people who live there and can be reflective of who they are. The same is true for outdoor public spaces. Gardens can include plants and flowers that have meaning to residents, as well meaningful items within them, such as benches or lines to hang clothing. Supporting the self in private spaces is a bit easier. Bedrooms can include photographs and other items that have meaning and are reflective of who the person is. The room décor could also be reflective of the person who lives there, and residents can be included in selecting items such as bedspreads and draperies. The same is true for bathrooms. These do not have to be cold, sterile, nonpersonal rooms. At the same time, they cannot be overstimulating or confusing. They can include personal items that reflect the person as well as items that provide a sense of home.

Identity and Home

Home is an important part of who we are. It is a reflection of our self. *Rethinking Alzheimer's Care* discussed the home in great detail, not only the place of home but, more importantly, the feeling of home. Brawley (1997) described how home is not just a place, but a concept of comfort and familiarity that nourishes the body and soul and that etches indelible memories in the mind. Home has also been described as "the experience of a fluid and dynamic intimate relationship between the individual and the environment" (Carboni, 1990, p. 32). Carboni also explained that the environment is made up of physical, social, and psychological spaces around the individual. The connections and interactions between the spaces and the individual provide a sense of identity that is essential in maintaining the self.

A few authors have described components of *being* at home, most significantly the relationships within them. Together, they help shape the experience of being at home. These components consist of meaningful relationships with oneself (e.g., inner self, calmness) and with others (e.g., spouses, relatives, friends, pets). They also include relationships with time (e.g., day, period in history), objects (e.g., photographs, furniture), events (e.g., chores, work, hobbies, school), and place (e.g., house, neighborhood, town) (Zingmark et al., 1993). It is a very integrated approach, where each component fits together to create the overall experience of being at home. Meaningful relationships with each of the components allow a person to fully experience being at home. The level of significance or importance of each component, however, varies from individual to individual.

Meaningful relationships are a fundamental component of being at home and impact the feeling of home. Of all of the previously mentioned relationships, those with oneself and those with others are of significant importance and deserve special attention. Beginning with relationships with oneself, being at home can be a very personal feeling, where an individual needs to *be* and feel at home with him- or herself before being at home or feeling at home with others. Through relationships with others, an individual may fulfill a need to have family connections, ties, and a clear identification of roles and responsibilities. Simply feeling the presence of others is as meaningful or even more meaningful than the interaction with others, simply knowing that someone is there. Meaningful relationships with others maintain a connection with things that are known and familiar, and allow an individual to be and to feel at home.

There are many elements of being at home that allow us to *feel* at home. Feeling at home and comfortable within our surroundings includes the presence of some elements and at the same time the absence of others.

A few authors have identified different elements of being at home (Zing-mark et al., 1995). Recognizing and fostering these elements are fundamental in supporting and facilitating the feeling of home for individuals with dementia. People must feel a sense of *safety* and *security*, while at the same time having the *freedom* to make choices, take risks, and be themselves. They must feel in *control* and have the *power* and *initiative* to do as they wish. In addition, there must be a sense of *order, possession, privacy,* and *recognition*. Individuals with dementia need physical and mental *nourishment*, a sense of being *rooted*, as well as a feeling of *togetherness, belonging,* and *connection*. Finally, they need to feel *joy* and *harmony*, that things known and familiar to them fit together and that good times can and do exist.

Understanding home can be challenging since each person's idea of home may be unique to and have a specific meaning to him or her, especially during certain periods of life. There are, however, some common elements mentioned above that are shared by all individuals that help foster the universal feeling of being at home. This feeling of being at home is what we must strive to truly capture and re-create in Alzheimer's care to support the self. The key is to recognize the differences in the many meanings of home and at the same time to celebrate the similarities.

Time must be taken to find out what home means to each individual and to learn about the many things that create the feeling of home. Individuals should be given the opportunity to help create their own environments—physically, emotionally, and culturally. Families can help by sharing stories and ideas of what home was like for the person with Alzheimer's. Staff must believe in, practice, and internalize this way of thinking and of lending support. Also, policies must reflect this philosophy of care and be developed with enough flexibility to sustain it.

The different components of being at home should be explored and included in care plans, such as accessibility to certain items, interactions with specific people, or taking part in specific events. Every effort should be made to identify those elements that constitute the feeling of home, and caregivers should continually strive to support and re-create them. As eloquently put by a person with dementia, "Home is when I'm with people I care about and who care about me."

Connections, relationships, and interactions with the elements of home are fundamental to the feeling of home. Care providers must move beyond the physical environment when attempting to re-create home and must better explore, understand, and support the emotional and cultural aspects of home as well. Only then can the feeling of home and how it can help support selfhood be truly understood.

Therapeutic Milieu and Dementia Care

In dementia care, all of the components of an environment must be considered since they form a framework for care that supports functional abilities, compensates for losses, and maintains the self. The concept of *milieu* is essentially the blending of the physical, social, and cultural environments. It recognizes the importance of the totality of one's experience. The concept is essential in caring for people with dementia because all of the elements of an environment are interactive and blend to form a whole that determines the kinds of experiences the person will have. In *Rethinking Alzheimer's Care*, Jane Stansell discusses the concept of therapeutic milieu in great detail. Part of that discussion is highlighted and expanded upon below to illustrate how a supportive environment can help to maintain selfhood. John Gunderson described five elements in a therapeutic milieu, which were adapted by Taft et al. (1993), for providing care for a person with dementia: safety, structure, support, involvement, and validation.

Safety

People with dementia need to be in a safe environment. The challenge is to provide safety in a way that it is not controlling. Milieu can be created to meet safety needs in many ways. For example, access to areas that could pose a danger can be limited and people can be engaged in meaningful activities so that they are not constantly being told, "No," "Stop," or " You can't go in there."

Structure

Structure is created for the person with dementia by providing temporal landmarks and a routine that offers predictability in the person's day as well as through the physical environment (Taft et al., 1993). The type and the amount of structure that may be helpful vary from person to person. For those who want and need structure and information, calendars, event listings, pictures, and verbal reminders are important. For others, these types of structured orientation are confusing and distressing. It is important to be sensitive to the kind and amount of structure that is really helpful. For people with dementia who have lost the ability to structure time, the structure of program activities is comforting. The routine of the day provides some predictability, a sense of rhythm and familiarity. At the same time, the routine of their own, typical day is reflective of and maintains the self.

Support

Support is conscious efforts to help people feel understood and to enhance their self-esteem (Taft et al., 1993). Intentionality is important in creating opportunities for people with dementia to feel competent and supported through activities appropriate to their abilities. Conscious effort in programs that provide care for people with dementia goes beyond the empathy and caring of staff and emphasizes the importance of thoughtful planning of activities and of taking deliberate steps to develop supportive relationships that are reflective of the whole self. Caregivers need to create a milieu where people with dementia feel supported by recognizing the importance of and fostering the development of supportive relationships.

Involvement

Involvement is engaging or interacting with our social environment (Taft et al., 1993). As social beings, we all feel the need to relate to others in a meaningful way. People with dementia feel the same need for social interactions. Sometimes caregivers become so focused on the mechanics of providing care that they lose sight of the reality of people with dementia. As the disease progresses, many people become less inhibited and lose some of their characteristic reserve when expressing feelings (positive and negative) in social settings. As the social façade fades, the person is able to interact with others in often more genuine and authentic ways than before. However, it is important to keep in mind that these enriching and reciprocal relationships can only occur if those providing care recognize the social needs of the person with dementia and accept the responsibility to meet those needs.

Validation

Validation is a process that affirms a person's individuality, feelings, and abilities. Behaviors are seen as meaningful and as a way of communicating, rather than as problems (Taft et al., 1993). The goal of a validation approach is to help the person maintain a sense of control in a situation, to facilitate the use of strengths to solve or cope with a problem, and to validate the person's worth. Providing a milieu that validates a person's individuality requires the development of a program that consistently affirms his or her unique abilities. Validation is not just provided by others, but is also the result of experiencing success in one's daily activities. Programs that are designed to use a person's retained skills and abilities provide multiple opportunities for validation.

Personhood as a Framework for Guiding Care

Chapter One discussed Tom Kitwood's work and the importance of personhood and person-centered care. Kitwood (1997) developed a conceptual approach to care that provides staff with a way of thinking about what they do according to the following 10 principles that guide care and that reinforce or support personhood and well-being throughout the course of dementia:

- Recognition
- Negotiation
- Collaboration
- Play
- Timalation
- Celebration
- Relaxation
- Validation
- Holding
- Facilitation

Rather than simply providing care in accordance with routines organized for staff convenience, efficiency, or some other criteria, Kitwood suggested that the focus should be on the person who is the recipient of care.

Kitwood's framework encourages staff to focus less on *what* is done and more on *how* it is done. It is almost as though the activities and communication strategies are vehicles that carry the real substance of care: care of the person and support of the self. Kitwood's principles assist those who provide care to critically evaluate how programs and communication strategies can be adopted and implemented to support the multidimensional person with dementia. This is in contrast with previous approaches to care that have focused, more narrowly, on custodial tasks or symptom management. Kitwood's principles provide us with a language to shape individual clinical practice as well as the means to develop this capacity within an organized program of care in a systematic and thoughtful way. They are described in great detail in *Rethinking Alzheimer's Care* and are discussed in this chapter because they provide an excellent framework for exploring our interactions in the environment and how they relate to the maintenance of self.

Recognition

Recognition is acknowledging the individual as the unique person he or she is. It includes verbal and nonverbal responses, especially direct eye contact. It may be a simple greeting or may involve careful listening over a period of time. Staff sensitivity is demonstrated when a form of acknowledgment is tailored to the individual and is consistent with the individual's unique capacity to receive and express a relationship with another. The art and subtlety should be reflected in staff's familiarity with that individual. Examples include saying "Hello, Professor" instead of "Hi, John" when you pass someone in the hallway who identifies himself with his years of teaching at a university, or referring to a woman as Grandma Jean instead of Mrs. Hulnick because it is how she was known by all of her neighbors.

Negotiation

Negotiation involves asking a person with dementia about his or her preferences, desires, and needs. This process should be a theme throughout the pacing of everyday activities as well as for individual situations that may arise. The key to negotiation is openness regarding issues that may not have been, historically, a matter of choice. An example of negotiation is consulting with a person and deciding on desired mealtimes or on what clothes to wear that day.

Collaboration

The collaboration approach requires a conscious choice to work with the person in partnership. Care is not done to the person as if he or she were a passive recipient. Collaboration can occur as a part of personal care, of specific projects, or in daily interactions. The care provider must gauge the comfort level of the individual by his or her responses to a conversation or to a care approach. The focus must include an appreciation of what the person with dementia wants or needs, apart from what staff may want or have as an agenda. Staff members must have a capacity to monitor their own body language and how others perceive or respond to them. For true collaboration to occur, staff must first be committed to the belief and value that the person being cared for is entitled to be a partner in decisions involving his or her care, and not merely a recipient or object of care. Many clinicians liken this process to a dance in which each partner must be sensitive and responsive to the other in order to coordinate and execute steps with a smooth and natural flow. Collaboration can take place while preparing a meal or while using the bathroom—when an everyday activity becomes a seamless partnership and we are *doing with* rather than *doing to*.

Play

Play involves spontaneity and self-expression for its own sake, with no particular goal in mind other than its intrinsic value and joy in the moment. This may be among the most difficult concepts for staff and families to appreciate and feel comfortable with. For most adults, the capacity to enjoy the simple events around us, with great abandon and glee, can initially be a bit unnerving. The ability to suspend logic is often a critical ingredient in caring for or in sharing enjoyable life experiences with a person with dementia. It is possible to have fun in the moment, to create fun or respond to situations lightly, and to share the humor as it presents itself. Examples of play include spontaneously singing a song, sharing a dance, or trying on a funny hat for a laugh.

Timalation

Kitwood (1997) coined the word *timalation*, a hybrid of the Greek word *timao* (I honor) and *stimulation*. This care approach emphasizes the use of the senses to interact and to provide contact, reassurance, and pleasure when other forms of interaction are less available to the person because of advancing cognitive losses. Some persons with diminished capacity to express or to understand verbal language may also have sensory impairment, which exacerbates the challenge of interacting with others. It is crucial that staff maintain communication through all other sensory channels that are available, to help the person maintain a connection to others and to avoid premature and unnecessary decline due to understimulation and withdrawal from people and activities. Aromatherapy or a simple massage are good examples of timalation.

Celebration

The intent of celebration is to share planned or spontaneous events without the concern of the artificial boundaries of the care-providing or care-receiving role. Using appropriate judgment, staff often can share a part of themselves with the individuals whom they care for and about. The key is to always monitor whose needs are being met in a situation and to ensure that an exchange is always in the interest of the person with dementia. Of course, honoring a birthday is an example of celebration, but so is sharing a special day with others, such as the first day of school for a grandchild. It is less about special occasions and more about sharing joyful moments.

Relaxation

Differentiated from other care approaches by the lowest level of intensity and the slowest pace, relaxation occurs when staff are involved and very much present with the person who has dementia. There does not have to be something going on, but there is the feeling of welcome, accessibility, and comfort. Relaxing interactions may occur during a lull in the schedule of more structured activities, at the beginning or end of scheduled events, or while en route on a day trip. This sharing time may not involve conversation, but should always include nonverbal communication that clearly conveys "We're together." This may be expressed in some form of touch or perhaps through a playful smile, wink, or nod—something sufficient enough to maintain or reinforce a sense of a shared and desired connection. Just sitting next to someone and allowing him or her to feel or sense your presence is often relaxing in nature.

Validation

Validation involves a high degree of empathy in the relationship in an attempt to fully understand and accept the reality and power of the other person's frame of reference, no matter how strange it might seem. This active acceptance is one of the most critical skills in caring for persons with dementia. The effort to *tune in* to what the person with dementia seems to be experiencing sets the stage for the types of communication and activities that staff can incorporate into its care approaches. Validation is in contrast to imposing a care approach by rote using information lifted from a book, pamphlet, or training video. It requires that the caregiver first appreciate who the person is, and from there selecting and modifying actions in accordance with what the individual seems to need most at a particular time. There is a sensitivity to timing and a nuance that create the *fit* between the general care approach and the specific tailoring of that approach to really fit the person and the circumstance. Validation requires that caregivers recognize, respect, and empathize with the feelings and needs of the person with dementia and what has become his or her reality. Observing and exploring the reality of a person with dementia and responding to a person's feelings and emotions with appropriate verbal and nonverbal techniques are examples of validation.

Holding

Holding essentially is being with a person, conveying a presence with and for the person in distress. It is an affirmation of support and answers an unspoken fear of abandonment. It gives the individual a grounding and centeredness that may be lacking when he or she feels overwhelmed with some emotion. In addition to encompassing the literal meaning of physical contact, holding must convey that the individual is not alone, that the caregiver is there with and for him or her. Success in using this approach is based on knowledge of the individual. Physical holding (e.g., a hug) may be the source of distress while at other times a possible means to alleviate distress.

When physically holding an individual, caregivers must be sensitive to feedback from the person. The expression of support may be more or less physical, depending on the individual's response to efforts to try and help him or her. At times a hug or an arm around the shoulder may be the support that is needed, while at other times providing a safe psychological space for or truly listening to and acknowledging the person is what is needed.

Facilitation

Facilitation enables the individual to accomplish what he or she wants and needs to do but cannot do independently because he or she is unable to initiate or complete the sequence of steps in an activity. The artistry of this approach is in supporting or supplementing the person's effort in a quiet way that is sufficient to complete the task at hand. The result is that the person feels a sense of satisfaction in having accomplished what was intended. Facilitation should be integrated into every interaction and care approach. It is fundamental to care that supports the self. For example, gently moving a slice of bread over a bit to be in line with the knife with butter that the person is holding is a simple action that facilitates success. Or handing a person a soaped-up warm washcloth and guiding the motion of face washing can facilitate a successful self-care experience.

Approaches to Care and Interventions

In the late 1990s, I was privileged to be part of research conducted by Lois Taft at the day center where I was working. Taft et al. (1997) described seven types of interventions that were identified from interviews with caregivers about the specific approaches to care that they provide:

- Social
- Psychological
- Functional
- Behavioral
- Environmental
- Medical
- Cognitive

These approaches are consistent with those described in Kitwood's framework and support personhood and well-being. They can be used as a framework to organize thinking about care approaches and interactions.

For experienced staff in everyday practice, these approaches are not usually part of a conscious process of selection. Often it is difficult to tease out the precise reason for responding in a given way. Typically, approaches serve more than one purpose and are often woven into everyday care. In caring for persons with dementia, it may be useful to try to think about the reason for selecting a certain way of responding to a person in a particular situation and to evaluate the effectiveness of the approach as well as the consequence.

Social Approaches

Social interventions encourage interpersonal interaction and social functioning. In daily care this would include activities aimed at supporting purposeful engagement with people and projects, relating to persons in dynamic ways that help the individual stay connected with those in his or her environment, and providing empathic caring and supportive touch. In addition to more traditional activity programs, there are many ways to encourage social functioning. For example, persons with dementia often yearn to be of service to others. Depending on individual capacities, this may include participating in the assembly of the community's newsletter or selecting or arranging materials for the bulletin boards.

Psychological Approaches

Psychological interventions recognize and support the individuality and the continued psychological functioning of the person living with dementia. Caregivers use these kinds of approaches when they: are responsive, see the world from the perspective of the person with dementia, offer choices, follow the person's lead, and reframe or explain a situation to enable a person to cope better with a given situation. There is a wide diversity in the human response to dementia. Many individuals with dementia are aware of their losses and, as with all human beings, express their feelings in words or through their behavior. Caregivers must try to be open to hearing and understanding this information, to providing persons with dementia the opportunity to share their concerns through words and behavior, and to providing the appropriate level of support.

Functional Approaches

Functional approaches promote physical functioning and facilitate as much independence with activities of daily living as the person is capable of doing. A caregiver's interventions may include providing direct assistance, cues, supervision, or rest periods. Staff and family must experiment with the best blend of assistance needed. Often subtle changes in individual staff approaches may elicit a different response. If more than one person provides care, it is important to be sure that they communicate with one another. It may expand or enrich the style of each care provider and may lead to better care for the person by offering the optimal assistance.

Behavioral Approaches

Behavioral interventions are nonpharmacological. They reinforce or promote desirable behaviors and alter undesirable behaviors. Examples of behavioral approaches include diversion, noninterference monitoring, going along with, time away, delaying tactics, and use of therapeutic untruths. Taft et al. (1997) elicited and reported caregiver behavioral interventions without commenting on or endorsing their merit. The author only supports the use of behavioral approaches that are supportive and truthful in nature and intent.

Environmental Approaches

Environmental interventions modify the physical environment to promote the safety and well-being of the person. Examples include modifying environmental stimuli, providing safety modifications, limiting access, providing personal identification, and using signage.

Medical Approaches

Medical interventions are pharmacological and are used to modify behavior, improve cognitive functioning, or maintain comfort. Although medical interventions may be helpful in many situations, researchers and clinicians believe that behavioral approaches should be considered as a first level of intervention before considering the use of medications. Many behaviors attributed to dementia may indeed be the result of medical problems that are avoidable and that can be remedied through more careful monitoring and management.

Cognitive Approaches

Cognitive approaches promote continued cognitive functioning and include reorienting and helping the person to remember. There are many opportunities for caregivers to assist those with dementia in staying connected to the world, by focusing on facts and by more generally noting landmarks of people, places, and events. It is important to gauge how the person responds to the facts and to be sure that you are meeting the individual's needs when trying to ensure orientation. In general, the emotional reality is more important than the temporal or factual reality.

Clustering as a Way to Organize an Environment and to Support Selfhood

Clustering people with dementia into groups with similar abilities and needs is a way to adjust all the components of the milieu to be supportive of the person with dementia. The physical, social, and cultural environment can be adapted to support the specific strengths and abilities of each person in a group setting. The milieu can also be designed to compensate for the specific losses of each group member by eliminating, to the extent possible, all the barriers that may prevent a person from using retained skills.

The concept of clustering is based on the belief that people with dementia retain their essence, core identity, and personhood throughout the course of the disease. It is an extension of the way most people live their lives. We all tend to have an affinity for people with whom we share interests and abilities. As a result of the disease process, many people with dementia lose the capacity to seek out others with whom they might share a rewarding and supportive relationship. Clustering is a means of compensating for that loss.

The impairment caused by the disease requires the help of caregivers to lessen the impact of the disease on the person's physical and psychosocial functional ability, including the ability to relate to others as a social being. Since the amount of support needed varies among people, and even from day to day with the person, it is necessary to carefully monitor the amount of support provided. Clustering people into groups with others who have similar abilities and needs makes supporting individual strengths and meeting individual needs possible without one-to-one staff–resident ratios.

Clustering is a means of organizing care and activities for people with varying abilities and needs based on current functional ability. It is a means of creating a more homogenous group for the purpose of providing activities and care that are a good fit for the person with dementia as well as of helping him or her to succeed in an activity, task, or interaction. Activities within clusters focus on process, are based on current interests, and are adapted to current functional level. Often, there may be individual activities taking place within a cluster.

Just as activities must be carefully adapted to match the core identity and functional ability of the person, so too must the interpersonal approaches used to engage the person in activities. Successful approaches are more often selected because they enhance a person's sense of him- or herself and because of appropriateness in a specific situation. Interactions focus on developing relationships and encourage individual engagement. Often the *how* is critically important, not the *what*. Subtlety in employing an approach or making an adaptation in an activity is essential. One must make a conscious and purposeful effort to provide assistance in a way that is not obvious and that does not call attention to a particular difficulty.

Clustering involves matching all of the elements of the milieu as closely as possible to the abilities and needs of the person with dementia. It is not about grouping people by disease classifications, by stages of the disease, or by mini-mental scores. Clustering is based on the person's predominant characteristics and abilities, not on a single impairment. It is based on the totality of a person's characteristics and carefully balances all of the person's strengths and abilities.

Providing Activities within an Environment

There are many specific care approaches and types of activities to use in caring for someone with Alzheimer's. This section does not provide a list of activities, but rather discusses them in a broad sense, the overall philosophy behind them and how they can be vital in supporting selfhood.

In the late 1990s, Melanie Chavin and I developed a national training program for the Alzheimer's Association called Activity-Based Alzheimer Care (ABAC). The program is offered through local chapters across the country and is designed to help care providers think about activities in a general sense to really impact how they work with individuals with dementia.

Chavin and I define *activity* as the interaction between an individual and the environment—physical, social, and cultural. Activities must be meaningful and appropriate. Meaningful activities reflect an individual's interests and lifestyle, are enjoyable to the individual, help the individual feel useful, and provide a sense of belonging. Activities are appropriate when they are meaningful for the individual and when they respect the individual's age, beliefs, culture, values, and life experiences.

An activity can be anything that is done throughout the day, not only what is scheduled and provided in a group setting. Activities should reflect the natural flow of the day for a person, which may vary from day to day and throughout the disease course. ABAC has four domains of activity: productive, leisure, self-care, and insightful. The program challenges trainees to take a look at their programs and be sure they are meeting their residents' needs in each of the domains. At the same time, it encourages care providers to really get to know the person with the disease and to develop a plan of care appropriate for that individual. The models discussed in Chapter One can be useful guides for getting to know a person and for choosing the most appropriate activities for the person. For example, the wellness model can

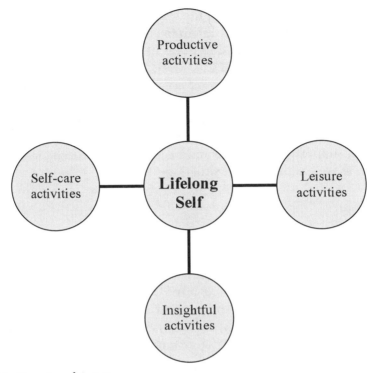

Figure 5.1. Domains of Activity

help staff to assess a person in six domains (physical, social, intellectual, emotional, spiritual, and vocational) and to build programs and interactions that are reflective of how the person identifies with each domain.

Activities need to be planned and organized and caregivers must be able to adapt them to an individual's needs and to daily situations. ABAC applies a concept called *flexible structure*, which is a method of organization that is responsive and adaptive to changes and needs. Flexible structure should also be used when creating activity schedules or calendars. Schedules and calendars should be flexible enough to be adapted to changing needs and situations. In a sense, the caregiver must be aware of how things are working and *go with the flow* to decide what will happen next.

Building programs and interactions around the concept of strength-based programming is key to the maintenance of self. Strength-based programming takes into consideration the individual's abilities, interests, and strengths rather than his or her problems, weaknesses, or losses. Whether in a mixed-group setting or in a cluster, finding ways to meet individual needs is key. For example, activity grading, which was developed by Jitka Zgola, allows individuals to participate in the same activity at different levels, from an observer to an independent organizer or doer. The activity or project is adapted based on the strengths and needs of different individuals so that all can be involved and can succeed.

The approach to or philosophy of activities within an environment is an important part of supporting the self. Activities must be appropriate, meaningful, and representative of the whole person—who he or she is now and who he or she has been throughout his or her life. Activities must also be flexible and supportive in nature and be adapted to the changing needs of the person as well as to different situations.

Closing

The environment is a key element of support in care that maintains the self. The physical environment can be organized to support continued functioning and selfhood, and care approaches and interactions can be carried out in ways that are reflective of person-centered care. Programs and activities must evolve over time to recognize and support the lifelong self of each person within the changing context of the disease. A supportive environment is the foundation of a care community that maintains selfhood in Alzheimer's care.

SELF-Reflection

CREATING AN ENVIRONMENT THAT SUPPORTS THE SELF

Calkins and Sloane (1997) described the following ten goals of environmental design in dementia care. Think about these goals and how your care environment is reflective of each of them. Introduce one or two of them at staff meetings and discuss them with others. Or, discuss them in relation to an individual as an example of developing an individualized care plan.

1. Maximizing awareness and orientation
2. Ensuring safety and security
3. Providing privacy
4. Supporting functional abilities
5. Adjusting the amount of stimulation
6. Providing positive quality stimulation
7. Providing opportunities for personal control
8. Facilitating social contact
9. Maintaining self-identity
10. Adapting to the stage of the disease

SELF-Reflection

PROVIDING PROGRAMS THAT ARE REFLECTIVE OF EACH OF THE DOMAINS OF SELF

Think about individual activities and group programs. Do they reflect the whole person and all of the domains of a person? Are they reflective of the whole self or of the lifelong self? What can you do to make them more reflective of either the whole or lifelong self?

Domains of Self

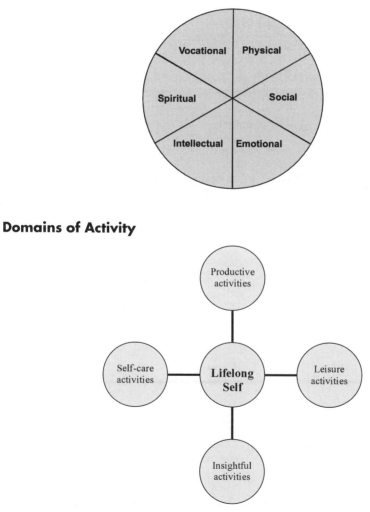

Domains of Activity

The Enduring Self in People with Alzheimer's. © 2008 by Health Professions Press.

SELF-Reflection

DESIGNING CARE APPROACHES THAT SUPPORT THE SELF

Think about your care approaches, either in general categories or specific types. Are they supportive of the self? Use Taft's overall model or Kitwood's more specific approaches and areas to think about the types of care that you provide in general or specifically in relation to one individual.

Taft's approaches:

Social   Environmental
Psychological   Medical
Functional   Cognitive
Behavioral

Kitwood's approaches:

Recognition   Celebration
Negotiation   Relaxation
Collaboration   Validation
Play   Holding
Timalation   Facilitation

CHAPTER SIX

RELATIONSHIPS AND INTERACTIONS THAT SUPPORT THE SELF

Umuntu ngumuntu ngabantu in Zulu conveys the idea that "a person is a person through others."

Sabat (2006)

Caregivers, family, and friends play an important role in maintaining or supporting the self in Alzheimer's care. Many researchers believe that relationships and communication are the two key components of person-centered care. Approaches to forming relationships, to listening and communicating, and to making connections can all have an impact on the self. This chapter describes how relationships are a vital component of care that supports the self.

Social Construction of the Self

Just as Tom Kitwood is fundamental to the discussion of personhood, Steven Sabat is essential to the discussion of selfhood and the impact of others on the self. Sabat, a neuropsychologist, has continued the discussion of Kitwood's beliefs and developed many concepts regarding selfhood and how others influence the self. His important work has strongly influenced my own research and writing. Sabat (2002) described the self of personal identity, how one describes him- or herself, and the self of social identity, or how one presents his or her identity to others. Personal identity is more internally focused whereas social identity is externally focused and dependent on the environment and interactions within it. Sabat and Harre (1992) asserted that the self of social identity can be lost indirectly as a result of how others treat and view the person with Alzheimer's disease (AD). Alzheimer's also

99

can affect the self of personal identity. Shenk et al. (2002) observed that the neurological impairments caused by the disease make it difficult for the individual to effectively organize and maintain his or her personhood and self-identity. It is important that interactions support the lifelong attributes of the self rather than focus on disease attributes. As with any new aspects of the self, the diseased self must be incorporated into the existing self. However, individuals with cognitive impairments are in a more vulnerable position than individuals without cognitive impairments, because they are particularly reliant on others to support and maintain selfhood.

Sabat (2006) discussed the concept of malignant social positioning in the context of conversational exchanges in which people take, impose on others, and reject or accept positions that make their actions intelligible as social acts. Sabat explained that positions help to define, strengthen, or weaken a person's moral and personal attributes and help to create story lines about a person. "Through the process of positioning, people explain their own behavior as well as that of others, so that to explain someone's actions in ways that emphasize the individual's negative attributes is to position that person in a potentially malignant way" (Sabat, 2006, p. 289). Sabat (2006) goes on to state that when a person negatively positions another, it is possible for the targeted person to reject the positioning being imposed on him or her. However, if the person who is being positioned negatively has dementia, he or she may not have the ability to make that rejection for a variety of reasons. Sabat (2006) continues,

> Thus, what is initially negative positioning can become malignant, or dangerous, because (1) the behavior of the person with dementia is increasingly interpreted in defective terms; (2) the person thus positioned is then treated as being defective so that 'malignant social psychology' ensues; (3) the person can then come to see themselves in progressively more defective terms and lose a sense of self worth; (4) if their behavior is negatively affected by ways in which they are treated by others, this possibility may go unnoticed and will continue; and (5) the dysfunctional relationship will continue to have a negative impact on the person with dementia and the results of that impact will be attributed to the disease and may generate a vicious cycle whereby the effects of the dysfunctional relationship are perceived as evidence validating the original negative positioning. (p. 290)

Negative positioning can lead to depersonalization of the individual. Kitwood (1990) described the following 10 processes and interactions that tend to depersonalize a person with dementia:

> *Treachery:* Some form of dishonest representation, trickery, or deception used by someone to get the person with dementia to comply with his or her wishes.

Disempowerment: Things are done for the person with dementia, even though he or she is able to do them in some manner.

Infantilism: An extreme form of disempowerment where the person is treated as a child.

Intimidation: The person with dementia is afraid of certain processes carried out in impersonal ways by powerful others, mainly professionals.

Labeling: A diagnosis brings expectations and sets up a self-fulfilling prophecy of those in decline.

Stigmatization: Similar to labeling but also carries connotations of exclusion.

Outpacing: Even though the person with dementia functions at a slower pace, those around him or her continue to move at a normal pace.

Invalidation: The person with dementia is ignored or overlooked.

Banishment: The person with dementia is seen as intolerable and removed from physical and psychological human interaction.

Objectification: The person with dementia is treated less like a person and more like an object.

Kitwood (1990) gave the following reasons as explanations for why some caregivers use malignant social psychology in dealing with the neurological impairment of a person with dementia:

- Many caregivers and service providers are extremely lacking in intersubjective insight.
- Caregivers are busy and face pressure.
- There is a tendency not to believe that the individual with dementia is a person, and so he or she is not treated with the respect that he or she deserves as a person.
- There may be some unconscious motives that engender a malignant social psychology.

What is key is that malignant social psychology is malignant because of the negative and depersonalizing effects on the person. In general, many caregivers function with goodwill, kindness, and commitment with limited resources and without malicious intentions. How caregivers respond to a person with AD, to the cognitive impairments caused by the disease, to his or her communication of distress, or to his or her inability to fully engage in social settings, may mean the difference between optimal person-centered care and the psychological invalidation of the person and of the self (Lipowski, 1969).

The Role of Others in Person-Centered Care

The role of other persons is essential in person-centered care or care that supports the self. Kitwood and Bredin (1992) discussed how interdependence is a necessary condition of being human. However, a dependence on others is forced upon people with dementia. The care provider becomes an absolute necessity, both physically and psychologically. This relationship is crucial. It is often the case that a person with dementia who is withdrawing or becoming demoralized is transformed by a little real attention and human contact. Kitwood and Bredin (1992) explained that personhood is not the property of the individual and can only be provided or assured within the context of a mutually recognizing, respecting, and trusting relationship.

Surr (2006) described a socio-biographical theory of self in dementia care in which interpersonal relationships with others, the broader social context, and the sharing of stories are important in maintaining the self. Knowledge of a person's biography helps in interpreting these stories. Surr (2006) found that the quality of relationships with family, other residents, and staff was particularly significant in either the preservation or undermining of self. Surr also discussed the work of other researchers who asserted that the development and maintenance of self is related to recognition and equality in interpersonal relationships, and that the loss of self occurs if recognition and equality do not exist in the relationship. This is especially true when individuals with AD are in situations that only allow them to receive and do not provide them the opportunity also to give.

The quality of an interpersonal relationship is colored by the person's perspective or view of the relationship. Ethicist Stephen Post has written about this topic in relation to what he characterizes as our *hyper-cognitive culture*—a culture in which the values of rationality, self-control, and mental and physical self-development are emphasized to the exclusion of all others (Ballenger, 2006). Post stated that our culture has the tendency to think that people with dementia lack any moral significance, that "We divide 'them' from 'us'; drawing a line between the rational and less rational, the unforgetful and the most forgetful, thereby exposing people with dementia to a vulnerability manifest in disregard of their remaining capacities, subjectivity, and well-being" (Ballenger, 2006, p. 162). Kitwood and Bredin (1992) also discussed the clear division that can take place between *us and them*, between those considered to be *normal* and those with dementia. Often, care providers believe that people with dementia are damaged and that they have a problem to be fixed. They are expected to come back to our world. Changes in such thinking are an essential component of the preservation of self for people with dementia and should be a crucial element in their care.

Relationships with others indeed have an impact on personhood. Kitwood and Bredin (1992) stated that the personhood of people with dementia needs to be continually replenished, their selfhood continually evoked and reassured. The other, the caregiver, is needed to offset degeneration and fragmentation and to sustain personhood. The further the dementia advances, the greater the need for *person-work*. The caregiver is needed to hold the pieces together, to become the memory. Kitwood and Bredin (1992) also maintained that this may be understood as the true agenda of dementia care. As care partners, we need to be the support that maintains the self and we need to structure the environment and interactions within it to effectively do so.

Relationship-Based Approach to Care

Relationships are key to good dementia care. Similar to other relationships in our lives, care relationships take time to develop and take effort to maintain and sustain. Some may be easier than others, and some may present many challenges. Others may bring exciting opportunities and wonderful gifts. All relationships are essential in dementia care. Care partners must find ways to make relationships work for those for whom they care. This process differs a bit from how relationships are developed and maintained outside of the care setting.

Relationships go through developmental phases. The first phase is one of getting to know each other. As we discussed in earlier chapters, time must be taken to really get to know the person with dementia. This often requires a bit more work on the part of the care provider because the person cannot always initiate interactions that reveal aspects of his or her self, particularly lifelong aspects. The next phase is the forming and developing of the relationship, which typically involves getting to know more about the person, his or her likes and dislikes, and the nuances of his or her personality. Trust and support are typically developed in this phase through interactions and shared activities. The final phase involves maintaining and evolving the relationship. Relationships typically have an ebb and flow to them, a give and take. There are great days and not so great days, but there is typically a commitment to sustaining the good of the relationship. Time and patience are often needed to understand and connect to the person with dementia and to truly be there for him or her. A caregiver's knowledge of the person, his or her attitudes about the person, and the interactions and activities that both share will all impact the relationship. All relationships require time to develop and a commitment to maintain.

A relationship-based approach to care is built around the concept that care takes place within a relationship and that the relationship is necessary for true person-centered care. There is reciprocity in the relationship, where both partners give and take. There is a commitment to getting to know the other, to sharing, connecting, and being with the person. Partners care about one another and are *available* within shared interactions. In dementia care, it becomes the responsibility of the care provider to actively find ways to support and maintain the self, both lifelong and current, of the person with dementia.

Building a Caring Relationship through Listening and Communication

People with dementia have difficulty expressing thoughts and emotions as well as understanding the thoughts and emotions of others. Many variables may affect the person's ability to communicate and understand, including disease progression, time of day, location, the other person, distractions, and stimulation. This section does not focus on specific strategies or techniques in communicating with a person with dementia. Rather, the focus is more on an overall philosophy of communicating within a caring relationship.

Goldsmith (1996) discussed ground rules regarding the attitude of mind that people must bring to the process of communication with people with dementia. Specific techniques and strategies do not matter if the overall philosophy is not there. Care providers must be able to listen, to accept the person as he or she is, and to be open to the possibilities of communication. At the same time, care providers must be able to look beyond the words and to observe the nonverbal ways people can and do communicate.

Seman (2002) defined meaningful communication as engagement on deeper levels that involves feelings and meanings that grapple with issues related to self-esteem, one's relationships with others, and one's place in the world. Meaningful communication requires others to *be with* the person with dementia, to give him or her undivided attention and emotional presence. This type of availability requires the caregiver to dedicate all of his or her senses to the person—to listen, to actually hear, to observe, and to demonstrate a connection to the individual. Meaningful communication involves acting as a facilitator. Seman (2002) continues, "It involves letting them know that they have been heard and trying to elicit what, if anything, is required of us—supplying a missing word, a hug, an empathetic response, information, a word of encouragement or hope, an honest answer, a laugh, a segue into another, less stressful activity" (p. 137).

Communication in a caring relationship requires that the care provider maintain a level of openness, attentiveness, and mindfulness that helps the person with dementia to be successful in communicating. Care providers must listen attentively, some say with a third ear, to seek out the emotional message or need, which at times may not be conveyed in words. They must also be emotionally available and must learn to show their availability both verbally and nonverbally so that the person being cared for recognizes and believes it. At the same time, care providers must take the time to observe and to adapt their manner of communication over time, as their knowledge of and as the needs of the individual being cared for evolve.

Caring communication is not about getting the correct answer, quizzing about the past, or using the right word. It is about truly listening and connecting. It is about looking at the situation from the perspective of the person with dementia. It is also about feeling the emotion and helping to convey the meaning of what he or she is trying to communicate. It is about being there in the moment and allowing the past to influence the present but not restrict or dictate it.

Goldsmith (1996) described communication as "more of an art than a science" and that you must "have a kind of poetic awareness" when communicating. Some describe it as similar to being an interpreter of a foreign language. The caregiver must be able to look for metaphor and allusion rather than specific meaning, must recognize the hidden meaning behind the words, and must try to get a *feel* for the essence or core of the communication. At the same time, Kitwood (1993) asserted that the caregiver needs to take on the role of a counselor or coach to keep the conversation open and allow and support the person to respond. For example, at the day center John asked where he could find the fish bowl. Since there were not any fish at the center, the staff member was confused about what John was looking for and thought it had to be something more. A few minutes later John was tugging on his belt and saying in a concerned tone, "I have to empty this thing." The staff member asked him if he needed to use the bathroom and John said yes. The fish bowl he was looking for was actually the toilet. In this situation, the staff member knew that John seemed very concerned and that the fish bowl was most likely representative of something else. The staff member took the time to really listen for the meaning behind the words and allowed John to communicate his need in the manner that he was able to at the time.

The caregiver must also learn to slow down his or her thought processes and become inwardly quiet. He or she must also adapt and slow the sense of time and pace to meet the pace of the person in his or her care, rather than expect the person to meet the caregiver's pace. Goldsmith (1996) agreed and noted that it takes time for people with dementia to get into the *communicative mode*. It also often takes time for them to process and understand communication. Rushing the communication does not help. It can take time, and caregivers need to devote adequate time to communication. Of course, time and competing demands are issues for many workers. Staff must, however, be able to deal with the pressures of time and find ways to work through them. Goldsmith (1996) recommended that training to build confidence in communication among staff is necessary. At the same time, a facility's management must allow and encourage time for staff to interact and employ the art of listening. Staff must be assured that it is okay to take the time to sit alongside a person with dementia and have a meaningful communication.

Nonverbal communication is particularly important, and is often overlooked. What is not being said can be more important than what is being said. Kitwood (1993) stated that people with dementia

> have a heightened awareness of body language, and often their main meanings may be conveyed nonverbally. In the case of those who are severely impaired in cognition, it seems probable that the words and sentences are at times more of an accompaniment or adornment than the vehicle for carrying the significant message . . . (p. 64)

Nonverbal gestures can often be ignored or dismissed, or go unnoticed by a caregiver when, in fact, they are important attempts at continued and meaningful communication. Caregivers must take the time to slow down, observe, notice, and support nonverbal types of communication. Jaber Gubrium described how a caregiver support group articulated a folk theory of dementia that rejects the notion that the self is lost with cognitive skills in favor of a view that an essential self remains intact, a self that can be reached by using nonverbal, noncognitive means of communication (Ballenger, 2006).

Meaningful communication is not a luxury, but rather a necessity. It should not be seen as only a means to the end of completing a care task. Rather, it should be seen as a beginning. It is the start of getting to know someone, sharing thoughts and insights, and learning to connect. It is the start of an opportunity to build and sustain deep and meaningful relationships with people with dementia as an essential part of their care.

Soulful Connections in Everyday Interaction and Care

Throughout my years of being in caring environments, I have found that many people with Alzheimer's disease experience and communicate from the soul. The disease process eventually forces them to live this way. They may retreat from an *intellectual existence* to a place of inner riches and spiritual freedom. In a sense, they can experience a reawakening or a return to a more genuine and authentic existence. They can connect on both a deeper and simpler level—heart to heart or soul to soul rather than mind to mind. Those who care for persons with Alzheimer's have the same ability, but may not necessarily realize it. Caregivers too often overlook these powerful, yet subtle connections because they become preoccupied with frustrations of loss and focus on what the person no longer can do.

The person with Alzheimer's has no other choice than to live in the moment. At times, past and future lose their significance and the here and now means everything. This allows persons with AD to take part in the ultimate existential experience—to be totally present with the moment. On other occasions, the uncommon blending of the past, present, and future shapes the now. Therefore, the way most of us live, with the chronology of time and with distinct compartmentalized segments of the past, present, and future, needs to be altered. This way of existence is an ongoing challenge for caregivers as they try to alter their own habitual ways of thinking and acting to become more open, flexible, and responsive to fleeting, ever-changing moments and events. If the moment means nothing later, in a sense it means everything now. The key is to allow the moment to happen, to share it, and to stay open to the possibilities.

The person with Alzheimer's also needs life to be simplified. At times, he or she may simply enjoy *being* with someone rather than constantly *doing* something. The end result is no longer as important as the process; presence means everything. This is a particular challenge for those interacting with a person with Alzheimer's when trying to make him or her complete tasks, insisting on a tangible end product, or participate in a *logical and purposeful* conversation.

People with AD also can let go of the ego and accept, relate, and connect with other people more authentically. Others are often seen without titles, labels, or skin colors—they are simply other individuals. Many times inner beauty is recognized and appreciated, and people accept one another without conditions. Many of us struggle throughout our lives to live free of prejudice and stereotypes and to allow ourselves to be open and compassionate with those who seem different.

Alzheimer's is also a catalyst for expressiveness, creativity, and emotional freedom. People with AD can become very passionate about their beliefs and concerns, and their passion may be misinterpreted as violence or anger. They can also appreciate humor, as they are able to take life and, at times, their everyday mishaps lightly. Grudges no longer persist because issues tend to disappear along with the moment. This can be a good example for many of us who take things too seriously and are often encouraged not to openly express our emotions.

Instead of trying to teach the person with Alzheimer's to come back to our chaotic and often preoccupied existence, caregivers need to stop and begin to encourage themselves to learn from those experiencing the disease. Everything that people with dementia experience is not bad all of the time. Caregivers must try to join them in their world, to model their behavior and interactions, and to allow them to teach us how to live more simply again.

There is more to Alzheimer's than loss and decline. However, we do not generally hear about it. The progression of loss and deterioration is also an evolution of growth and development, an evolution that many never have the opportunity to experience because we deny it to ourselves and to the person with the disease. Instead of looking at everything that is being taken away, we need to begin to look at what is being given to us—an opportunity for soulful thoughts, experiences, and connections. Again, this is what many struggle to achieve throughout their lives. We must recognize these *soulful* times and be present with them. In short, the opportunity for caregivers to nourish their souls is reinforced daily by the person with the disease, who is the essence of a soul on its journey.

It is important that care providers learn to recognize and cultivate the soul in Alzheimer's care. Care providers are key to deeper connections, interactions, and relationships that support the self. The presence of Alzheimer's disease can offer many opportunities of the soul—experiences, connections, and actions. Think about times when you have seen or interacted with someone with Alzheimer's, a family member, or even a fellow care provider when things seemed somewhat different, yet more significant or powerful. These can be the times when we acknowledge the soul, either deliberately or by chance. A few examples follow:

- Times when you have felt totally connected with a person with Alzheimer's and when you saw that connection in the person's eyes or face or even felt it in your heart.

- When you knew a person's need without exchanging a word, or knew how to respond without ever having interacted with someone before.

- Times you were lost in the moment when interacting with someone with Alzheimer's.

- Situations when you allowed yourself simply to *be* with someone with Alzheimer's and focus on what he or she felt was important or meaningful.

- Experiences when you felt the power and soul of touch in a care situation.
- Situations when you felt the pain, embarrassment, or frustration of a person with AD.
- Times when a person with Alzheimer's was able to sense something was bothering you when friends and colleagues could not notice.
- When you were part of a *magical moment*, but you could not describe or felt funny describing it to others.
- Situations when you saw two people with Alzheimer's relating in a different or special way.

Ballenger (2006) described how one caregiver felt the disease brought her closer to God. The caregiver's belief is based on the concept of soul or spirit. Although the spirit remains intact in dementia, a society that confuses intellect or function with the true essence of self fails to recognize this. Ballenger continues, "Alzheimer's strips away the characteristics we use to identify one with the world, leaving the spirit of the person intact. It is that spirit that is able to respond to love and knows the comforting presence of another" (Ballenger, 2006, 156).

Ballenger (2006) also shared a story of a woman who was caring for her husband who believed that the self does remain in dementia, that dementia does not destroy the true self, but in fact helps to reveal it. The wife stated that her husband was much closer to his feelings and basic instincts, much like other individuals with dementia and less like so-called normal individuals. Ballenger explained that, "In the process of becoming civilized and formally educated we often become separated from our feelings and skeptical of our instincts. We put our trust instead in written and visual information, purportedly proven by someone else" (Ballenger, 2006, 158). Ballenger continued: "The definition of a person is to be found in the relationship between the definer and defined" (Ballenger, 2006, 160).

Authors, family members, care providers, and individuals with dementia have begun to discuss what the disease gives to them rather than only what it takes away. They have identified opportunities for positive experiences, for natural evolutions and resolutions, for personal growth and development, and for deep connections and relationships. For instance, a daughter I knew described how she was able to have a very different and fulfilling relationship with her father since she started caring for him. She mentioned that he worked a lot when she was younger, and that as a young adult she went through some difficult times and would fight a lot with him. She was so thankful for their time together and their new connection.

In regards to relationships, many family members and caregivers have identified the following positive opportunities:

- to share memories and experiences from an earlier time
- to express caring through adapting
- to experience surprises and excitement
- to love unconditionally
- to *be* together
- to share physical and emotional closeness
- to experience a nurturing role
- to relate to a loved one on a soulful level

These types of *real* connections are at the core of care relationships.

Closing

The role of others in maintaining selfhood in people with dementia is quite significant. Caregivers must take an active role in supporting and maintaining the self of persons with Alzheimer's, which includes creating environments and activites that help and encourage the person to stay involved, to communicate, and to connect. A relationship-based approach to care allows caregivers to get to know the person and then to structure interactions that support the lifelong and current self and that result in optimal functioning of the person. Caregivers must learn to connect, to allow themselves to be in the moment, and to communicate and listen with intention. Finally, as care evolves, caregivers must stay flexible and evaluate and adapt the care approach as necessary—all in an effort to sustain meaningful relationships that maintain the self.

SELF-Reflection

FACILITATING INTERACTIONS RELATED TO SIX DOMAINS OF SELF

Think about the types of interactions that would support the self in the six domains of self. Some examples are provided below to get you started.

Physical—opportunities to participate in self care or exercise

Emotional—opportunities to share feelings or be an outlet for stress

Intellectual—opportunities to solve problems and make decisions

Social—opportunities to be or not be with other people

Vocational—opportunities to use life skills and expertise

Spiritual—opportunities to attend a service or be alone with thoughts

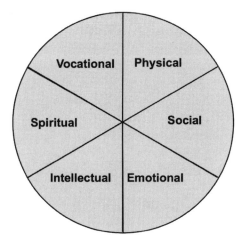

SELF-Reflection

COMMUNICATING IN WAYS THAT SUPPORT THE SELF

Instead of providing specific strategies, this chapter discussed general themes in listening and communicating that may be helpful. Think about ways that you communicate with individuals with dementia. How are you doing in each of the following themes? What can you do differently?

- Listening actively and attentively for meaning
- Being available and present
- Slowing down
- Observing and listening nonverbally
- Demonstrating connection
- Facilitating interaction or exchange of information

At the same time, think about factors that may influence communication, such as disease process, time of day, location, personal style, distraction, or stimulation.

SECTION III

KEY CONCEPTS FOR
MAINTAINING THE SELF

CHAPTER SEVEN

SUPPORTING THE SELF IN EVERYDAY CARE

We must allow the past to influence the present, but not to restrict or limit it.

Sam Fazio

As was discussed in the previous chapters, good person-focused care means finding ways to support the self in everyday care and interaction. It requires that the caregiver know the person as well as focus on caring about and building on strengths and abilities. It also requires the caregiver to be in the moment, to foster relationships, and to build programs that are reflective of the self of the person being cared for. This chapter ties together the previous chapters and translates the concepts discussed in each into everyday applications—all in an effort to maintain the self in Alzheimer's care.

Maintaining a Sense of Self

Some researchers have begun to examine and discuss how individuals with Alzheimer's maintain their sense of self throughout the disease course. Pearce et al. (2002) conducted a qualitative study that examined the appraisals and coping processes of individuals diagnosed with early-stage Alzheimer's disease (AD). Semi-structured interviews were conducted with men who had AD and with their wives who cared for them, which resulted in several themes. Their findings suggested a circular and ongoing process in which men attempted to manage their sense of self by balancing their wish to maintain a prior sense of self against their need to reappraise and construct a new sense of self. This idea is similar to what was discussed in Chapter Two regarding the evolving self through adulthood.

The men's attempts to maintain a sense of an existing or prior self in the context of dementia was represented by the following seven themes:

- *Limited impact:* The men tried to limit the impact of the disease on their everyday lives and functioning.
- *Normal memory loss and aging:* The changes were viewed as part of normal brain aging.
- *Try a bit harder:* The men engaged in active efforts to work/perform to their previous standard.
- *Take a break:* Breaks were taken from trying to remember something or complete a task.
- *Make the most of things:* An effort was made to make the best of things and get on with life the best they could.
- *Reliance on wife:* The men relied on their wives for both emotional and practical support.
- *Reliance on medication and services:* Outside resources were viewed as a vital attempt to maintain a sense of self.

The men's attempts to reappraise and reconstruct a new sense of self with differing expectations and roles was represented by the following seven themes:

- *Loss:* Expressed some degree of loss
- *Change over time:* Continually reappraised their abilities and reconstructed differing selves
- *Uncertainty:* Indicated some degree of uncertainty about the future
- *Awareness of difference:* Expressed that their own perceptions differed from their wives
- *Concern for partner:* Expressed concern for wife—losses, lifestyle, health
- *Difference:* Considered their memory difficulties to be worse than others
- *Downgrade expectations:* Began to reappraise their abilities, relationships, and roles

Clare (2003) continued the work and found that people fell along a continuum between self-maintaining and self-adjusting. Those on the one end interpreted situations as normal in an effort to maintain continuity of a previous self, and those on the other end found ways to incorporate the dementia into the formation of a new sense of self. It is important to support the maintenance of selfhood and self-identity so as to optimize the personal resources available for ongoing coping and adjustment (Downs et al., 2006).

Supporting the Evolving Self

Key to maintaining the self is learning how to support the evolving self. It is important to connect with who the person is currently, to support who the person has been throughout his or her life, and to stay open to exploring who he or she is becoming. The past must be allowed to influence the present, yet not to define it. The present must also be allowed to influence the present. At the same time, both the past and the present must be allowed to shape the future, and the future must be left free to influence itself. This may sound a bit confusing; however, very simply, we must not allow ourselves to be restricted by the past and have expectations grounded solely in past performance and perceptions.

As discussed in Chapter Two, a person's self evolves as he or she develops with age and over time. At the same time, experiences and other factors impact the evolving self and affect the various dimensions differently for each individual. New components of the self need to be appropriately incorporated into the existing self, such as an illness or a disease. The new component becomes a part of who the person is, but not all the person is. Those who do not have cognitive difficulties incorporate new components of the self into the existing self on an ongoing basis. However, those with cognitive difficulties may not have that ability. Caregivers must be sure to see the person for who he or she is now as well as for who he or she has been throughout his or her life, and not just in terms of his or her illness or symptoms.

In some cases, a new component of the self may not be exactly what was expected or was typical of the person before onset of the disease. Caregivers must remind themselves that a new component, whether it is what was expected or not, is a part of who the person is becoming. Once a caregiver accepts the new component of the self and connects with it, the care experience changes for everyone. Some believe that a new or different part of the self may have always existed but that social pressures and masks concealed it. The loss of inhibition associated with Alzheimer's may allow the new component to surface and, in a sense, may also allow the person to develop a freer and truer self.

Creating a Prosthetic or Supportive Environment

A prosthetic environment is a supportive environment that compensates for one's losses or weaknesses and builds upon one's strengths and abilities, all in an effort to allow for optimal functioning and success. Just as a prosthetic leg can allow someone to walk, a prosthetic environment can allow a person with dementia to be successful and to maintain functioning, whether it be in an activity of daily living, such as bathing, using the toilet, and dining, or in communicating interests, needs, or aspects of the self.

The level and type of support that is provided to the individual is very important. The support goes beyond modifications in the physical environment and is more about the specific interactions that take place within the environment that allow it to be supportive. Developmental psychologist Lev Vygotsky developed the concept of the *zone of proximal development*, which represents the difference between the actual developmental level of a child and his or her potential development with assistance, guidance, and supervision from an adult collaborator or peer. This concept is grounded in the belief that children can accomplish tasks or solve problems beyond their current ability with assistance. Related to the zone of proximal development is a concept called *scaffolding*, which occurs when *experts* are sensitive to the ability of a *novice* and respond in a supportive manner to the learning situation so that the novice gradually increases his or her understanding and ability (Bjorklund, 2000). Barbara Rogoff viewed this interchange as an *apprentice in thinking*, where novice children improve their skills and understanding through participation with more skilled partners in culturally organized activities (Bjorklund, 2000). Rogoff developed the concept of *guided participation* as an extension of Vgotsky's zone of proximal development. Guided participation is the process of involving individuals with others as they communicate and engage in shared activities (Bjoorlund, 2000).

Some practitioners have begun to consider adapting the concept of guided participation to people with disabilities and even cognitive impairments. Specifically related to older adults and person-centered care, Mather LifeWays Institute of Aging developed a strategy called Just Right Challenge for use in one of its training programs. Just Right Challenge is a technique for supporting a person's independence and success and for finding the right balance between what a person can do for him- or herself and when he or she needs help. I refer to this type of involvement within a prosthetic environment as *supportive encouragement*, which provides the support an individual needs to maintain or improve his or her abilities and functioning while at the same time encouraging him or her to accomplish the most he or she can do to be successful. All of this is done with the lifelong self in mind. Care partners must continually find ways to supportively encourage people with dementia in everyday care and interaction, allowing them to function at their best and to continue to stay involved, as appropriate.

Providing a prosthetic environment for memory and aspects of lifelong self is also essential. Sometimes the caregiver has to become the memory for the person with dementia. Often, the caregiver must keep the memories alive, but it needs to be done in a way that is supportive and that helps to maintain the self. The caregiver needs to fill in the blanks and to be an assistive or supplemental memory. It is important not to quiz the person about the past or specific facts, but to provide additional information or reminders to allow the person to be successful in maintaining his or her self—current and lifelong.

Creating a prosthetic environment also means weaving everyday choices into the broader practice of empowerment. Many individuals with dementia are not heard and their wishes are not taken into consideration; however, practice has shown that most people can express their choices and needs and can be active partners to varying degrees. Care providers need to listen, observe, interpret, and support this type of involvement in everyday care and interaction. Empowerment involves not only offering choices but also respecting them. Choices such as what to wear, when to eat, or which chair to sit in are important. Having a choice about whom to sit next to or choosing to be involved in an activity or not are examples of moving toward empowerment (Goldsmith, 1996). Creating opportunities for empowerment requires caregivers to expand their thinking about choices and autonomy.

The effects of not being included can be detrimental. Goldsmith (1996) discussed Rosemary Lubinski's description of the condition of *learned helplessness*. This occurs when a person perceives that events and outcomes are independent of his or her responses, so he or she comes to believe that any further action is pointless (Goldsmith, 1996). When a person with dementia thinks that his or her responses do not make a difference or are not heard, he or she simply stops responding. Goldsmith adds, "When this happens, then the significant people around them do not expect the person to provide direct feedback, or to be able to perform capably, and the vicious circle of dependency is reinforced and the person is disempowered even more" (Goldsmith, 1996, p. 66). It basically becomes a spiraling process of low expectations and high dependency. Goldsmith (1996) maintained that the more we appropriately expect from those with dementia, the more opportunities we will provide for them to respond and participate—and, ultimately, the more we will support the maintenance of self. Similarly, severe disability can occur when the physical and social environments create demands that exceed an individual's abilities, thus resulting in impairments that are disproportionate to those expected from their cognitive impairment. It is imperative that individuals are involved in appropriate ways so that they can continue to thrive and function and not experience additional impairments beyond what is considered typical.

Experiencing Flow

The expression *go with the flow* is probably familiar, but perhaps less well known is the concept of *flow*. Flow is the mental state that someone experiences when he or she is fully immersed in doing something, and it is characterized by a feeling of energized focus, full involvement, and success in the process of the activity (Csikszentmihalyi, 1990). Being *in the flow* is to be truly absorbed in an experience or activity. This may be the best definition of *connection* in dementia care—when one is fully involved in the moment. This notion is addressed in Chapter Six with the discussion on soulful connections.

Csikszentmihalyi (1990) identified the following components of an experience of flow: clear goals, concentration and focus, a loss of feeling of self-consciousness, a distorted sense of time, feedback, balance between ability level and challenge, a sense of control, intrinsic reward, and an emergence of action awareness. However, not all of these components are needed to experience flow. Caregivers cannot force flow to happen, but they can structure environments and interactions in ways that allow flow to emerge. It is next to impossible to experience flow in dementia care without also being able to *go with the flow*—although they mean different things. Caregivers must be flexible enough in their thinking and behavior to allow *what might be* to happen as well as to find ways to connect through flow and to experience all that flow has to offer.

Being in the Moment

Some Zen beliefs are helpful in approaching dementia care and in experiencing connections. An essential part of caring for someone with Alzheimer's disease is being able to embrace or *be* in the moment. But what does that really mean, and how can a caregiver realistically accomplish it, especially when there is so much going on within a care setting or when things are not exactly as they may have been expected to be?

It may be helpful to begin by describing the moment and why embracing it is so essential in Alzheimer's care. The moment is the present time, the current reality, or the here and now. It is what is happening, or even what could be happening, right now. The moment is always here, but it is also always changing. In a sense, we are always experiencing a brand new moment. It is somewhat paradoxical—it is here, yet gone; simple, yet complex; same, yet different. The moment represents a finite amount of time, but at the same time it is filled with infinite possibilities. These possibilities and the moment they exist within are fundamental components of good Alzheimer's care.

As mentioned in the discussion on soulful connections, people with Alzheimer's have no other choice than to live in the moment. So, as one man said, "If the moment means nothing later, it means everything now." Past and future begin to lose their significance and the present means everything. This type of existence, or living in the moment, can be extremely challenging for caregivers when the present seems so different from what the past was or what the future was going to be. However, there are ways to overcome those challenges and to embrace the moment—by allowing the past and the future to shape the moment, rather than sadden or limit it.

The present may be different than what was hoped for, but that does not have to be seen as all bad. The moment can be a wonderful place filled with many events never experienced before. It can also provide opportunities to connect with someone in ways never allowed before. In the moment, one can experience simple, more genuine interactions that allow for connections in authentic ways, rather than solely mind to mind.

Three Phases of the Moment

Embracing the moment consists of three phases. First, you must find the moment. You must then be able to experience it, or *be* in the moment. Finally, you must be able to find your way back to the moment so that you can experience it again in the future.

Finding the moment is not difficult, but it can be challenging. The moment cannot be forced or orchestrated, and staying open to it or being in the right place mentally can be a very conscious choice. Attention to the moment can be deliberate, but it cannot be intentional. It can be purposeful, but not planned. Very simply, the moment just happens—if you let it.

Experiencing the moment once it is found really requires a certain amount of flexibility or openness. Besides paying attention to it, being in the moment requires you to really clear your mind and to *go with the flow* or where the moment takes you. Many times, that means doing things differently or doing different things than before—things that may seem somewhat ridiculous, child-like, or even purposeless. The thing to remember is that they have purpose and meaning within in the moment, especially for the person with Alzheimer's.

Getting back to the moment or finding the moment again involves remembering what worked and what did not, what was done differently, and what *place* you were in. However, keep in mind that what worked one day may not the next day; this can be especially true for AD. Each moment is different and filled with a variety of possibilities. The challenge is to find the moment again and to allow yourself to be there with your experience and the person. Returning to a moment does not mean doing the same things again, but rather being in the same *place* again so that you can be open to going with the flow and to experiencing the moment and all that it has to offer. Remember, the *what* that happened in the moment is less important than the *how* that facilitated the *what* to happen.

Making the Moment a Caring Moment

The *how* is really what makes a moment become a caring moment. The specific steps to take or techniques to use are far less important than the reasons for creating a caring moment. The underlying philosophy of why caregivers do what they do is the foundation of a caring moment. The interactions that exist in the moment are all individualized and based on the person's needs, interests, strengths, and abilities. The interactions are key to a caring relationship and are all based on individual connections—connections that allow the possibilities of the moment to unfold. The following example illustrates how a moment can become a caring moment by being in the right *place* and letting it happen.

Allan had always been a particular man. He had his own way of doing things and often told others how to do things the "right" way. That's probably what made him such a good supervisor when he worked for the city of Chicago. His strong work ethic carried over to other parts of his life, including his time at the day center.

Allan's daily experience at the center was sometimes frustrating for him, especially when other participants in his group did not follow his directions and "do their jobs." Staff also found following some of Allan's directions to be a bit challenging from time to time. He often came across as being difficult, uncooperative, and bossy, which definitely influenced how he was perceived and approached by others.

One typical morning, Allan had some paper and a pencil and was telling others what needed to get done. He was becoming increasingly frustrated because people weren't doing what he had asked them to do and if they were, they weren't doing it correctly. On a nearby wall, a travel poster was losing its adhesiveness and was slowly coming down off the wall. As anticipated, Allan immediately told me to go over and fix it; however, I was busy working with another group member.

Allan decided that the only way to get the job done right in the first place was to do it himself, so he got up and attempted to fix it himself. However, he didn't seem to have the right equipment to complete the job correctly. His frustration with the situation and lack of appropriate tools was making him want to leave the room. I tried to divert his attention to other tasks; however, doing so was just leading to more frustration and anxiety. He needed the appropriate tool to complete the job correctly.

I purposefully decided to stop what I was doing, to go with the flow, and to help Allan find what he needed to complete the task. He and I then embarked on a perilous journey to find the right equipment to fix the falling poster. Outside the door of the group was a shelving unit filled with many odds and ends. Allan quickly looked around to try and find the right equipment for the job. When he found what he needed, a paint roller, Allan shouted, "There's that little bugger!" He then proceeded to lead me back into the group, directly to the falling poster, and began to show me how to appropriately get the job done. He very carefully and meticulously moved the paint roller over and over the poster, ridding it of every wrinkle. I assisted him and listened as he shared his expertise and stories with me. I quickly saw how his feelings of frustration were turning into ones of accomplishment as one of his workers (I) was finally doing the job correctly, and, more importantly, under his guidance. Throughout that morning, and in many days that followed, we continued fixing posters throughout the room together, as well as many other jobs that needed to get done.

The connection happened only because I became open to it and went with the flow of the moment. It allowed me to see another side of Allan that helped me to find ways to connect with him in the future. I shared some time with him on his terms, not mine; in his reality, not mine. The connection taught me a lot about caring in the moment, and how an interaction can help to support and maintain the lifelong self.

Narrative, Life Story, and the Maintenance of Self

How the story of self is created, re-created, and continually supported is also fundamental in maintaining the self. Psychologist Dan McAdams is an expert on identity and life story. As discussed in Chapter Two, McAdams asserted that a person's sense of identity is based on a story of how the person came into being, where the person has been, where he or she is going, and who he or she will become. He explained that people create a life story that is an internalized narrative with a beginning, middle, and anticipated ending. It is created and revised throughout adulthood as a person changes and as the changing environment places different demands on a person. According to McAdams, each life story contains consistent features, and the model for change in identity over time is the process of fashioning and refashioning one's life story (McAdams, 1993).

Surr (2006) explained that a narrative theory of self recognizes that the succession of one's life events becomes a coherent whole story that forms the basis of self, and that a person rewrites his or her life story throughout time. New experiences and situations are continually integrated into the story, and memories of the past are constantly reconstructed. An objective or factual account is not re-created, but rather reconstructed from selected events and experiences based on individual interpretation (Surr, 2006). This is key. As long as the individual sees an event or experience as fact, then it is. It should not matter if it is not necessarily true.

Anne Basting, director of the Center on Age and Community at the University of Wisconsin, through the StoryCorps Memory Loss Initiative, is very active in using storytelling in caring for people with dementia. Through her work, people with memory loss are supported and encouraged to share their stories. Her TimeSlips project encourages people with memory loss to continue to exercise their imaginations and creativity. At the 2006 Alzheimer's Association Dementia Care Conference, Basting discussed how she views the concept of reminiscence: that it is not about remembering specific details about the past, but rather putting memories (real or not) together to make a story. It is the weaving together of experiences. As the story is being created or told with another person, it is the process of engagement that is important. The story itself is what is most important, not the specific facts within the story. Psychologist Steven Sabat's work is also representative of the importance of the story itself, or of owning the pieces of it. Sabat and Collins (1999) discussed that the persistence of personal identity could be measured by the continued use of personal pronouns. It did not really matter whether the statement was factual or not, but rather that the statement was owned by and perceived as true for the person. The research study discussed in Chapter Four also examined personal pronouns as a representation of self.

Surr (2006) summarized the literature on the story of self and stated that there are three main types of story used in maintaining the self: (1) development and telling of a life story, (2) storied reconstruction of selected biographical life events and experiences, and (3) telling of metaphorical stories. Goldsmith (1996) discussed different approaches to life story, such as autobiography, oral history, reminiscence, and life review. Although there are subtle differences in the approaches, the outcome is the same. Life story can tell us information about the past that can be helpful in care and in interactions that maintain the self. It can tell us about lifelong patterns of communication and behavior, as well as about history, preferences, and insight. Life story can also give the opportunity to engage with someone and to get to know his or her self. It is the process of developing, telling, and reconstructing the life story and not the outcome that is important. Surr (2006) wrote that biographical theories suggest that narratives, life history, and their expression through the telling of stories are important elements in the development and preservation of self. Care providers must find ways within a care setting to keep life stories alive and to be sure others have access to them. This may be accomplished in a variety of ways, such as by creating life history books and audio or video recordings, or by engaging the residents in larger storytelling projects. The creating, knowing, and sharing of these stories are key in providing care that recognizes and supports the self.

Identity and Interventions

Other researchers are examining how aspects of the self or how identity roles can influence the development of care programs and interventions. Cohen-Mansfield et al. (2000) explored self-identity in individuals with dementia through structured interviews and case studies. They explored four types of role identity: professional, family-role, leisure activities, and personal attributes. They found that self-identity can change throughout dementia, with family roles retaining the greatest prominence in the present. They also asserted that self-identity can be used to improve quality of life. In a later study (2006) the researchers explored the salience of self-identity in the same four areas as perceived by individuals themselves, family members, and staff. The family role was found to be the most important and salient role identity, according to all three groups. Roles related to being a spouse, parent, or grandparent seemed most significant among individuals with dementia.

Cohen-Mansfield et al. (2006) explored the retention of these self-identity roles and their potential use in designing individualized interventions. Participants in the experimental group engaged in activities that corresponded with their most salient identity roles. The researchers found that the participants showed a significant increase in interest, pleasure, and involvement in activities and that they exhibited fewer agitated behaviors and increased orientation during the period. This study shows evidence that individualized interventions based on self-identity contribute to well-being. The researchers concluded that individualized interventions are not cost-prohibitive and can occur in small group settings or, at times, with minimal staff involvement.

It is important for caregivers to learn about an individual's lifelong self and identity roles and their significance as well as to develop programs and services that are supportive and reflective of that significance. It is also important for interactions, relationships, and interventions to be reflective of the aspects of self that are meaningful and significant for the individual.

Closing: An Illustration of Care that Maintains the Self

This section weaves together all of the discussions in this book regarding person-centered care using a real-world example. The story of Maria Rose Ventrezio illustrates how to create environments, programs, and interactions that are reflective of and that support the whole person and lifelong self. It will hopefully encourage you to take a look at your community to be sure that you are doing all that you can to get to know the self and to build care partnerships that support and maintain the self.

Getting to Know the Person

Maria Rose Ventrezio was born in Philadelphia on August 8, 1930. Her parents were both born in Italy and met in Philadelphia, where they raised their family. Maria has three brothers and two sisters, all of whom are still living but live out of town. She speaks to them regularly and is often visited by her siblings and her nieces and nephews when they are in town. Family has always meant a lot to Maria and gatherings have always been the norm for this Italian group of individuals. Traditions have been very important. Maria met her husband Salvatore in Philadelphia and moved to Chicago soon after they were married. Salvatore died about five years ago of a heart attack. They have two children, one son and one daughter, and five grandchildren. All of them live in the suburbs of Chicago. They typically visit on the weekends, when possible.

Maria mostly worked in the house as a homemaker and raising the children. From time to time, she was involved in some part-time work, such as a receptionist in a local dentist's office and as a helper in a day care center. She was also actively involved in her children's school and extracurricular activities at the park district. Maria has always enjoyed cooking and learning new skills in the kitchen. At the same time, she enjoyed reading fiction novels. She and her family traveled around the United States, and she always enjoyed those family trips. She has also enjoyed playing cards with her family and friends. Nowadays, Maria enjoys doing simple word-search puzzles, reading magazines, watching television, crocheting, and playing cards. Maria was raised as a Catholic and still participates in Sunday services and other religious traditions.

Maria has always been a good communicator and enjoys talking with other people. These days, she often has difficulty recalling words but can participate in conversations and can communicate her needs, although sometimes she needs assistance. She likes to spend some time in her room and also time in common areas talking with others and participating in programs. She often gets overwhelmed and anxious when too much is going on in the environment. She is in good health, with some arthritis in her knees and hands. Maria can get around the care community on her own but can become confused in finding her way back to her room from time to time.

In getting to know Maria, we talked with her, her family, and other staff. We also observed Maria in different situations and interactions. Using the six domains of a person and the seven attribute categories, we were able to gain a picture of Maria's lifelong self and current self. Some of the information we learned from Maria was different than the information from her family, which is okay because that is how Maria sees herself today. At the same time, some information that was provided by the family gave us additional information about Maria. For instance, she had a daughter that died in her teens and she does not like talking about it at all.

Maria's typical day before coming to the care community consisted of getting up early and sitting in the kitchen drinking coffee and reading the newspaper. She would then have a light breakfast and do some housecleaning. Her daily soap operas were often playing in the background, and she sat down to watch them from time to time. Sometimes, neighbors would stop over to visit or her son would come and visit. In the afternoon, she would often take a walk through the neighborhood or to the grocery store. She would sometimes work in the garden or do some knitting. Dinnertime was often a lonely time for Maria unless a friend or family member visited. In the evening, Maria would watch television—detective shows were her favorites—or read a book. She would often fall asleep in the chair and go up to bed around 10:00 p.m. The weekends would be a bit different, with more time in the yard, visits from children and grandchildren, big Sunday dinners, and card playing.

Relationships were very important to Maria, especially with her family. She also enjoyed relationships with neighbors and close lifelong friends, or "gomads" as she called them. However, many friends had died and others were difficult to visit. She talked often on the telephone with those she could.

Creating the Environment

When Maria moved into the care community, it was important to create an environment that supported her self. Maria was comfortable with living in a shared room because she enjoyed being around other people. She did enjoy her time alone though, so the room was organized so that there were separate areas for each person. The person she shared a room with was also a social person, and they seemed like a good match. Maria brought many items from home, including her bed and dresser, her favorite chair, and many personal items, such as photographs and knick-knacks. Maria was included in the process of decorating the room, from deciding where to place her items to selecting curtains and wallpaper for the room.

Some of Maria's personal items were also included throughout the care community, with the permission of her and her family. Some afghans she crocheted were included in the family room, some photographs were placed on common walls, and some other items were placed in a curio cabinet in the community room.

Maria's room entry was personalized with her name and with a collage of photographs. Her room and bathroom were organized to be supportive of her strengths and abilities, allowing her to use her retained skills and to maximize her functioning. Her room was at the end of the hallway, so that she would not be overwhelmed by the activity in the social area. Every effort was made to be sure that the physical and social environments were reflective of Maria's identity. These will continue to be assessed and adapted as needs change. The environment represented a therapeutic milieu that provided safety, support, structure, involvement, and validation, not only in the physical surroundings but in the relationships within the environment.

Fostering Supportive Care Approaches and Interactions

As the staff build relationships with Maria, many of Tom Kitwood's care approaches are helpful, such as recognition, collaboration, play, celebration, relaxation, validation, and facilitation. In their interactions and care approaches, staff members keep in mind that Maria is a social person and that relationships have specific meaning for her. Self-care takes place in collaboration with Maria so that she can continue to function successfully. Daily interactions take into account Maria's lifelong self and she is involved and engaged, as appropriate. Daily conversations and exchanges include information regarding her family, cooking, and Italian traditions, to name a few examples. Because Maria has some communication challenges, the social environment provides the support she needs to feel comfortable and successful in communicating. Since Maria has always been a social person and continues to be, interactions support appropriate involvement and participation in a variety of ways.

The care community finds ways to support Maria's typical day. For instance, staff allows her to come into the kitchen area early in the morning in her housedress to have a cup of coffee and read the paper. Then, after she returns to her room to get dressed for the day, she comes back into the dining room for breakfast and sits with other people she enjoys being with. As the day progresses, Maria is encouraged to make choices as to how to structure her day to be as reflective of her typical day as possible.

Building Appropriate Activities and Programs

Maria has opportunities to spend time during the day as she has done throughout her life. Her typical day in the care community did not have to be significantly altered regarding activities. Maria can choose which programs she wants to participate in. Those that match her lifelong self are encouraged, such as a travel group or intergenerational group. Also, a crocheting group and card-playing group were organized in the care community and take place on a regular basis. Since Maria enjoyed traveling so much, outings and armchair travel groups are good activities for her from time to time. She also has time alone to complete simple word-search puzzles, read, and watch television. Maria helps staff prepare meals from time to time, and helps in the cleaning of her room on a daily basis. In addition, there is a room available for Maria so that she can visit with her family members in private, or even so that she can share Sunday dinners together with them on occasion.

All of the six domains of self are represented in the activities Maria has the opportunity to be involved in. For instance, Maria can take part in walks, make choices and express concern, build social relationships, and continue to do puzzles. At the same time, Maria has the opportunity to participate in religious services and traditions and can continue her vocational work by helping around the care community with cooking and secretarial work. Maria is encouraged to participate in groups that are made up of individuals who have similar strengths, interests, and abilities as she has and the activities are representative of all domains of activity, not only the leisure component. Approaches and interactions within the activities are structured so that staff can supportively encourage Maria to be involved to the best of her ability and to continue to function at her optimal level. At the same time, staff allow possibilities to emerge out of the moment and are able to go with them as new possibilities present themselves.

Sharing, Evaluating, and Adapting

The process was not over once information about Maria had been gathered, approaches structured, and programs developed. Maria's life story continues to evolve and grow, and the care community actively supports that process. It is shared with others in the community on an ongoing basis and becomes a *living* document that evolves and changes with time, need, and situations. At the same time, Maria's life story influences care decisions and discussions throughout the entire disease process. It is a constant and ongoing reminder for providing person-centered care to Maria that recognizes her entire self and for finding ways to support and maintain herself in all interactions, care, and programs.

SELF-Reflection

USING ZEN PRACTICES TO EXPERIENCE THE MOMENT

Consider the following Zen practices to help find and experience the moment. These practices may not only be helpful in care interactions, but also in other aspects of your daily life.

Breathe deeply. Take in a deep breath and let it out. Feel your chest rise and fall as the air flows in and out. Concentrate on your breath and how your body and mind begin to respond to it.

Clear your mind. Focus only on the present. Put other things behind you. Forget about what you just completed or what you have to do next. Let go of anything that is frustrating to you.

Become attentive to the present. Begin to pay specific attention to things around you. Notice everything, yet focus on nothing. Use all of your senses.

Go with the flow. Let yourself become free and open to the moment, letting it guide your thoughts, actions, and interactions.

Connect with the person and experience. Relate to the person you are with and the experience you are a part of. Engage in a different type of activity, explore a new relationship, or simply try being instead of doing.

Stay open to the possibilities. Be willing to experience new opportunities and ways of doing things as the moment continues to unfold.

Shape future interactions. Allow your experience and relationship in the moment to shape future experiences and interactions.

SELF-Reflection

MAINTAINING THE SELF IN DAILY INTERACTIONS AND CARE

Think about how the self can be maintained in everyday care and interactions. Start with the following categories and examples and then add others. It may be helpful to think of other examples that are self-limiting and ones that are self-maintaining or supportive for each category. You may even want to discuss as a team or to consider categories and examples in relation to specific individuals in your care.

Mealtime
Self-limiting: Set times, undesirable food, assigned or inappropriate seating

Self-maintaining: Flexible times, food choices and preferences, choice of seating

Bathing
Self-limiting: Done to/for, open environment, cold, staff talking with other staff

Self-maintaining: Collaborative, warm temperature, privacy, staff talking with the person

Dressing
Self-limiting: Not based on lifelong style, no choice, hospital clothing, done for

Self-maintaining: Based on preferred style, choice, collaborative

Using the toilet
Self-limiting: Done for or told, pulling off clothes, staff talking to other staff

Self-maintaining: Collaborative and assistive, asked, reminders and prompts, staff talking with the person

Activities
Self-limiting: Only group activities, only based on perceived leisure, no choice in attendance

Self-maintaining: Based on individual interests, group and alone, choice in attendance, reflective of all domains

Support groups
Self-limiting: Negative- and problem-focused, not inclusive or flexible

Self-maintaining: Solution-focused, empowering, focus on remaining strengths and abilities, inclusive in nature

SHARING THE SELF WITH OTHERS

Inside yourself or outside, you never have to change what you see, only the way you see it.

Thaddeus Golas

This chapter provides a framework for sharing information about maintaining the self with other staff within your care community. It will hopefully save you some time and provide a springboard for discussion as you motivate others. As you know, some changes are easy, while others can be a bit more difficult and take time and attention. At the same time, people can get stuck in old, comfortable ways of doing things and can have many excuses for why things need to be or to stay the way they are. It is important that you be supportive, informative, and patient as you function as the catalyst for change.

Taking Action toward Change

The discussion that follows outlines steps that you can take to learn about maintaining the self in person-centered care, to share that information with other staff in the care community, and to be the agent of change within the community. This outline may prove to be helpful as you think about how to implement change within your community. It is not meant to be all-inclusive, but rather a framework for thinking about next steps. As with any plan, it is important that you make it your own and be sure it is appropriate for your community.

Review Materials and Resources

You will want to begin by refreshing yourself on the concepts presented in this book. You may even want to read some additional resources to be sure you have a solid grounding in the fundamentals (see the Recommended Readings). Take your time and really think about the concepts and how they apply to your community. Let the concepts ignite ideas of your own. At the same time, think about how you can continue to learn about maintaining the self in person-centered care. Be sure to find ways to stay on top of new materials and resources.

Meet with Leadership

With any new idea or program, it is important that the leadership within your community is in agreement. This can be a big challenge for many. Sometimes leaders become immediately concerned about increased budget and staffing, and it becomes your responsibility to explain how changes can take place with minimal cost and no additional staff. This is where you have to be creative and convincing, and where you have to become the *champion for change.*

Begin by sharing what you have learned from this book and from other resources. Highlight the key points and do not get caught up in all of the details; you can follow up on them at another time. Illustrate how change can have an impact on your care community. Be specific and point out the *win-win* opportunities. Talk about current operations as well as about what is working and what may be able to work more effectively or in a different way. Be sure not to point fingers; instead, emphasize what will make the most sense for the individuals in the community. After you discuss the importance of making change, decide upon next steps together. You may even need to identify some steps in advance and show that you have thought things through and are committed to this movement. Although difficult, buy-in from leadership is key to success.

Develop an Action Plan

You will need to have a plan for how you will implement within your community what you have learned. It can be as simple or detailed as you wish. The most important thing is that you take some time to think through how you will make things happen. At the same time, you will want to include others in the process so that they feel they are part of the development and implementation of the plan. You may even want to put an advisory team together to create and monitor the plan.

You will want to be sure to have both short-term and long-term goals. Be sure to set S.M.A.R.T. goals—specific, measurable, attainable, reasonable, and time-based. Identify specific strategies for accomplishing your goals. At the same time, think about possible challenges or barriers and how you might overcome them. Think about the resources you might need, too. Be sure to consider no-cost, low-cost, and high-cost options—whichever makes the most sense for your community. Finally, think about how you will track progress and measure success.

Share the Learning

It is important that you find ways to share what you have learned with others throughout your community who have a variety of roles and responsibilities. You will also want to be sure that the information is presented in nonthreatening and nonaccusatory ways. Also, be sure to keep in mind how adults learn and include real-life examples whenever possible. Remember that people generally want to know "what's in it for me?" or "how will this change my work?"

You may need to consider a variety of approaches to sharing what you have learned. Consider one-to-one coaching sessions or ongoing mentoring. Weekly team meetings are another avenue for presenting and discussing ideas. More formal in-service programs can provide information within a more significant block of time. Finally, a formal training session designed and delivered by staff or by an outside trainer can be organized to devote a day or half day to new learning. It is important to think about what will work best and meet the needs of the workers within your community.

Reward Change and Celebrate Success

Be sure to build a system to reward staff for changes in behaviors or patterns and for making change. This step is an important step that is often forgotten. In addition to creating a system that would allow managers to recognize the success of staff members, consider a system that would also allow staff to recognize each other. Think about giving low-cost or no-cost rewards beyond paper certificates. You may even want to have a monthly celebration and bring in a simple snack. Again, whatever will work best for your community.

Build a Support System

Without a support system in place, often the best plans can fall to the wayside. In the beginning, everyone is excited about the plan and is making changes. Then other priorities come up or barriers get in the way and the plan is put aside or simply given up because it seems too difficult or overwhelming. It is important to put in place a support system for yourself and for others to talk through challenges with one another and to share solutions. You may need to have a group of people within your organization, or even outside your organization, to provide ongoing support as you make changes. Care workers will need the same type of system to discuss daily struggles, to identify solutions, and to celebrate successes.

Evaluate and Revise

No plan is perfect and will need to be revised with time, new information, and experience. Be sure that you have a system in place to evaluate and revise your action plan as needed. Stay open to new ideas and to making changes when necessary. Others may come up with ideas that you may not even have thought about. Your advisory group may be useful in this process. You and they can review progress on an ongoing basis and decide upon revisions together.

Sharing Key Points with Other Staff

The following is an outline of key points from each chapter and provides some suggestions on how to share that information with others. It is provided as a general framework for you to build upon. You may want to explore some of the topics and not others—whatever makes sense for you and your care community. You may even want to make them into a slide presentation or handouts. A summary of the SELF-Reflections presented in each chapter is also provided for your reference. You may want to share these with other staff to stimulate discussion and action and to illustrate translation from concept to practice.

Learning is an ongoing and dynamic process. Sharing what is learned is just as important as the learning itself. This is especially true for information that can change thinking and caring, and that can change the culture of a caring community to recognize and maintain the self. As you learn and share, remember that simple changes have rippling effects.

Chapter One: The Self as the Core of Person-Centered Care

Person-Centered Care—Key Points to Share

Four key components of person-centered care (Brooker, 2004):

- Value people with dementia and those who care for them.
- Treat people as individuals.
- Look at the world from the perspective of the person with dementia.
- Provide a positive social environment in which the person with dementia can experience relative well-being.

Share the four key components outlined by Brooker (2004) to begin a discussion about person-centered care. Use Kitwood's theories to lay the foundation for a discussion about what type of care affirms personhood.

Culture change and the Pioneer Network:

- Culture change is a process—moving from a dependence-based model to an independence-based model focusing on autonomy and sense of control.
- Pioneer Network—nonprofit organization—is changing nursing home culture.

Highlight various culture change models. Review the Pioneer Network values and discuss how actions and interactions need to change to reflect those values.

Principles of caring:

- Caring requires us to care for the person, not the disease.
- Caring involves more than simply providing care.
- Caring shifts the focus from correcting to connecting.
- Caring involves listening for meaning.
- Caring requires us to communicate *caring* in our everyday care.
- Caring requires us to foster a caring community.

Share the descriptions of caring from Swanson and Callahan as background and to encourage discussion about what real caring looks like. Review the core values in providing care and use them to discuss what types of interactions and environments recognize and support these values.

Getting to know the person:

- More than a tool; a philosophy and process
- Get to know the *essence* of the person
- Multi-dimensional approach
- Include past and present characteristics
- Typical-day, relationship-based, and I-focused approaches
- Variety of sources and moments in time
- Build ways to share *stories* with others to impact care

Getting to know the person with dementia is the first step in providing care that recognizes and maintains the self. Discuss conventional and unconventional ways to get to know the person with dementia.

SELF-Reflections:

- Providing care that affirms personhood
- Using new words to describe Alzheimer's disease and the person
- Getting to know the entire self and creating a person-centered plan
- Getting to know an individual through assessment

Chapter Two: Overview of Self

The Self—Key Points to Share

Defining self:

- Self is the knowledge, feelings, and attitudes we have about our own being as unique functioning individuals (Lemme, 1999).
- Duality—inner and outer, private and public
- Influence of others

An overview of the self can be useful to engage in a discussion about what self means to each team member. Discuss how others are key in the formation of self and, more importantly, in the maintenance of self.

Evolving self through adulthood:

- New aspects added as one grows and develops
- Adapts to new environments and situations
- What we imagine ourselves becoming

It is important to talk about how the self is initially formed in childhood and continues to develop throughout the life course, even in adulthood. Share some of the theories related to this development. Also, encourage discussion about how adaptive the self can be when faced with new situations or experiences.

SELF-Reflections:

- Examining what self means to you

Chapter Three: Overview of Alzheimer's Disease

Alzheimer's Disease—Key Points to Share

Alzheimer's facts:

- 5 million people have Alzheimer's disease (AD) in the United States
- 1 in 10 have a family member with AD, and 1 in 3 knows someone
- Estimated that 16 million people will have AD by 2050
- Progressive, degenerative brain disease
- No cure, some treatments that slow progression and alleviate symptoms—more in the pipeline
- Nonpharmacological treatments shown to be effective

Share some general facts and statistics about AD. If needed, provide an overview of AD: warning signs, progression, diagnosis, and brain changes.

Stages or phases:

- Progression is very individual
- Various stage theories
- Prefer phases and suggest strength-focused model for person-centered care

Discuss stages or progression of AD and focus on a strength-based care model. Discuss other observed strengths as a group.

New models and ways of thinking:

- Holistic
- Person-centered
- Strength and ability-focused
- Relationship-based

Share some of the fundamental elements of innovative care models that are around today, as well as how thinking is changing in how we view the disease and the people who have it.

SELF-Reflections:

- De-medicalizing the approach to care
- Examining myths about Alzheimer's disease

Chapter Four: Evidence of the Self in Alzheimer's Disease

Evidence of Self in AD—Key Points to Share

Overview:

- Portrayals of AD often diminish the self.
- Self in AD has been measured through visual self-recognition and narrative techniques.
- Study conducted by author applies both methods, quantitatively and qualitatively.

Discuss how AD is often portrayed and how it can lead to damaging the self. Provide background by sharing some research highlights related to self and AD.

Study conducted by author:

- Participants: 78 English-speaking older adults divided into three groups—mild impairment, moderate impairment, and no impairment
- Materials: MMSE, FAS test, interview guide, and photographs
- Approach: individual meetings that were videotaped, coded, and analyzed

Share some information about the study, including who participated in it, what was used, how it took place, and how it was analyzed.

Key findings of study:

- Individuals who were more cognitively impaired overall used fewer attributes and pronouns.
- Individuals across all three groups used a similar rate of pronouns and attributes per minute.
- Proportionally, the types of attributes used were similar across all three groups.
- Themes of what individuals discussed were similar across all three groups.
- No major differences in visual self-recognition across the three groups.

Highlight the key findings of the study. You may want to use some of the charts or graphs in the appendix to illustrate key points and outcomes.

Implications on care:

- Self does persist and needs others to support/maintain it
- A prosthetic environment can support the self
- Recognize life-long self in environments and interactions

Facilitate a discussion about what evidence of the self means in relation to care and interactions.

SELF-Reflections:

- Thinking about the persistence of self

Physical and Social Environments—Key Points to Share

Ten goals of environmental design (Calkins and Sloane, 1997):

- Maximize awareness and orientation
- Ensure safety and security
- Provide privacy
- Support functional abilities
- Adjust the amount of stimulation
- Provide positive quality stimulation
- Provide opportunities for personal control
- Facilitate social contact
- Maintain self-identity
- Adapt to the stage of the disease

Rather than discussing physical environmental modifications, spend some time discussing general themes in design. You may also want to share the themes outlined by Cohen and Weisman (1991).

The meaning of home:

- More than just a *home-like* look—physical and psychosocial features
- Meaning of home is different for each person
- Care setting must capture being and feeling at home

Spend some time discussing the meaning of home, and how to create that feeling within your care setting.

Care approaches:

- Components of a therapeutic milieu, or the blending of the physical, social, and cultural environments to produce safety, structure, support, involvement, and validation
- Kitwood's 10 principles of person-centered care
- Taft et al. (1997) care approaches: social, psychological, functional, behavioral, environmental, medical, and cognitive

Use some of the general principles or approaches discussed in this chapter to facilitate a discussion about care within the environment.

Activities and involvement:

- Clustering—grouping individuals based on retained skills and abilities
- Meaningful and appropriate activities
- Multidimensional approach based on domains of a person
- Strength-based programming

Finally, spend a bit of time talking about programming and how it can be organized and implemented to support selfhood.

SELF-Reflections:

- Creating an environment that supports the self
- Providing programs that are reflective of all the domains of self
- Designing care approaches that support the self

Chapter Six: Relationships and Interactions that Support the Self

Relationships—Key Points to Share

Influence of others on self:

- Self can be lost indirectly as the result of how others treat and view the person with AD.
- People with AD become reliant on others to support and maintain self.
- Interactions must support lifelong self and not be limited to disease or symptoms.

Share some of the research on the influence of others on the self, specifically the work of Steven Sabat and his general themes in his findings. Also, encourage discussion by describing Kitwood's (1990) aspects of malignancy.

Relationship-based care:

- Relationships influence personhood.
- Person-centered care requires a relationship-based approach.
- Get to know the self and incorporate aspects of the self into everyday care and interactions.

Share the fundamentals of a relationship and discuss why it is important in care that supports the self.

Listening and communicating:

- Less about techniques, more about overall philosophy or approach
- Requires being present with the person
- Must truly listen and be open to the possibilities
- Look beyond words, including using nonverbal forms of communication

Rather than focusing on how-to lists for communication, facilitate a broader discussion about what it truly means to listen and communicate in care that maintains the self.

Soulful connections:

- Connect in genuine and authentic ways
- Deeper connections when the mind is uncluttered and open to new opportunities
- Living and being in the moment
- Opportunities for personal growth and development

Encourage a discussion about what it feels like to connect on a deeper level. Allow team members to share their thoughts and experiences.

SELF-Reflections:

- Facilitating interactions related to the six domains of self
- Communicating in ways that support the self

Chapter Seven: Supporting the Self in Everyday Care

Maintaining the Self—Key Points to Share

Evolving self:

- Balance maintaining a prior sense of self with constructing a new one.
- Allow the past to influence the present, but not to define or restrict it.
- Stay open to characteristics of the current self.

This last section should be used to tie everything together and to reflect on how thinking and acting need to change to support or maintain the evolving self. Clare's (2003) model may be helpful to set the stage, followed by a discussion of how the self evolves throughout the life course and based on situations and experiences.

Prosthetic environment:

- Compensates for losses and builds upon strengths and abilities
- Supportive encouragement—provides the support to maintain functioning while encouraging optimal success
- Compensates for memory and aspects of lifelong self
- Inclusion and empowerment

Spend some time talking about how the environment and interactions within it need to evolve to be supportive of strengths and abilities as well as of the self.

Being in the moment:

- Experiencing *flow*
- Phases of the moment—finding the moment, experiencing it, and finding the way back
- Make the moment a caring one

Explore the concept of being in the moment and discuss what it means for your community. Share an example of a moment that became a caring moment to illustrate the point.

Identity and interventions:

- Importance of life story and narratives
- Adapt programs and interventions as influenced by the aspects of self
- Care that maintains the self

Finally, discuss how specific interactions and programs can be adapted to meet the needs of an individual's current and lifelong self.

SELF-Reflections:

- Using Zen practices to experience the moment
- Maintaining the self in daily interactions and care

RESEARCH METHOD AND RESULTS

Overview of Study Method

Participants

Seventy-eight English-speaking older adults (ages 66 to 103) were recruited for the study. The majority of participants were Caucasian females with a high degree of education. Based on the Mini-Mental State Examination (MMSE) (Folstein et al., 1975), participants were classified with no cognitive impairment (MMSE 27–30), mild impairment (MMSE 21–26), or moderate impairment (MMSE 11–20). At each level of cognitive impairment, half of the individuals resided in the community and attended an adult day center and half were in a residential facility. Participants with cognitive impairments were diagnosed (by a physician and as identified from their chart) with probable Alzheimer's disease (AD) or an unspecified related dementia, and, as indicated by primary care providers, they had adequate language abilities and no serious co-existing health conditions that would affect their participation in the interview.

Research volunteers were recruited through several eldercare organizations in the greater Chicago area. After meeting with facility directors, potential participants were identified and introductory letters were shared with the individuals and their family members. Consent forms were given to unimpaired participants and to family members of cognitively impaired individuals. For the latter group, agreement was obtained at the first meeting. All participants were treated in accordance with the ethical principles of the American Psychological Association (2002).

Materials Used

The MMSE (Folstein et al., 1975) was used to index cognitive impairment and the FAS test (Borkowski et al., 1967) was used to assess verbal fluency. A semi-structured interview and discussion guide was used to stimulate discussion of self and to elicit the use of pronouns and personal attributes. Questions were developed to encourage the participant to discuss him or herself in relation to the following seven attribute categories based on Sabat and Collins (1999) and Sabat and Harre (1992):

- Physical traits
  - Lifelong
  - Disease-focused
- Personal characteristics and qualities
  - Lifelong
  - Disease-focused
- Familial
- Vocational or professional
- Educational
- Talents, hobbies, and interests
- Attitudes and beliefs
  - Lifelong
  - Disease-focused

The guide progressed from general and nonthreatening questions, such as "Tell me about yourself" and "How would you describe what you look like?," to more specific questions, such as "What is your philosophy of life?" and "What do you hope for and dream about?" If needed, a general probe of "Anything else?" or a targeted probe of "Can you tell me more about ____?" was used. The interview was videotaped.

Self-awareness was also observed by using self-recognition photograph test measures, which were adapted from various approaches employed in previous research (Biringer & Anderson, 1992; Grewal, 1994; Povinelli, 2001). Each participant's photograph was taken with an instant camera. In the individual test, each participant was shown his or her own picture and was asked, "Can you tell me who the person is in this photograph?" In the group test, each participant was shown a group of five photographs. One was the person's own picture taken earlier in the visit and the other four were of strangers of the same gender and similar age. The participant was asked, "Can you tell me which of these photographs is you?" Responses were recorded as correct or incorrect based on whether the participant recognized him- or herself.

Procedures

The study's lead investigator met individually with each participant on one occasion. Within each facility, meetings took place in a room with minimal distractions. The investigator explained the purpose of the study and obtained appropriate consent. The investigator administered the MMSE, took a photograph of the participant, and administered the FAS. Approximately three minutes later, the investigator asked the participant to identify the person in the photograph taken earlier (individual test) and then conducted the interview. Following the interview (which lasted for roughly 15 minutes on average), the participant was asked to identifiy him- or herself in the group test.

Coding

Videotaped interviews were transferred to mpeg data files, and Noldus The Observer software was used for coding. The lead investigator coded all interviews using a pre-established coding scheme. Pronoun use was coded by the use of *I, me, my, myself, mine, implicit* (e.g., "brown hair"), *plural* (e.g., "We have two children"), and *placeholder* (e.g., "I don't know" or "I think so"). Attribute use was coded using the seven categories mentioned earlier: physical traits; personal characteristics and qualities; familial; vocational or professional; educational; talents, hobbies, and interests; and attitudes and beliefs. Both *disease* and *lifelong* types of attributes in the categories of personal characteristics and qualities, physical traits, and attitudes and beliefs were also coded. An independent observer coded 25% of the interviews in each group, and was in agreement 88% of the time.

Results

Language Data

Total Frequency Usage. As hypothesized, there were differences in the frequency of pronoun and attribute use across levels of cognitive impairment, that is in the total number of times participants used pronouns and attributes in their interviews. A multivariate analysis of variance (MANOVA) was performed to assess the effect of cognitive impairment on total frequency of pronoun use and total attribute use. The overall MANOVA was reliable, $F(4, 148) = 9.54, p < .01, \eta^2 = .21$. Both frequency of pronoun use and attribute use declined significantly across levels of cognitive impairment. Mean frequencies of pronoun use were 114.6, 86.8, and 62.9 for those with no impairment, mild impairment, and moderate impairment, respectively. For attribute use, the corresponding means were 110.1, 75.3, and 55.2. In summary, individuals who were more cognitively impaired used fewer attributes and pronouns.

Production Rates. Since the total frequencies are mostly affected by cognitive and language deficits (i.e., total language abilities decline along with cognitive abilities), we sought a more appropriate measurement of self-knowledge (i.e., free of non–self-related constraints) by analyzing the rates of pronoun and attribute use. Rates were calculated by dividing the total number of pronouns or attributes by interview duration. As seen in Figure A.1, the mean numbers of pronouns and attributes produced per minute were very similar across the three levels of cognitive impairment. Statistically speaking, the MANOVA was not reliable, $F(4, 148) = 1.20$, $p = .31$, and the univariate tests also revealed no significant differences across levels of cognitive impairment in either pronoun or attribute use rates. In summary, individuals across all three levels of cognitive impairment used a similar number of pronouns and attributes per minute.

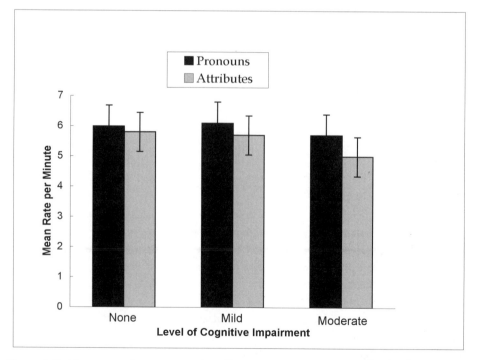

Figure A.1. Mean rate of pronoun and attribute use per minute across levels of cognitive impairment (bars indicate 95% confidence intervals).

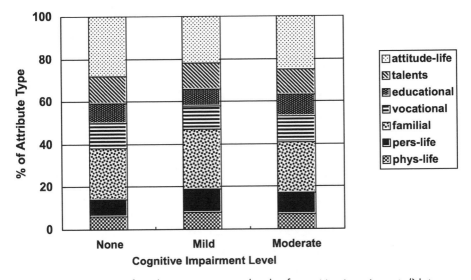

Figure A.2. Proportion of attribute types across levels of cognitive impairment. (Note: *attitude-life* = attitudes–lifelong attributes; *talents* = talents, hobbies, and interests attributes; *pers-life* = personal characteristics–lifelong attributes; *phys-life* = physical traits–lifelong attributes.)

Proportional Analyses. The proportion of attribute use per each of the seven categories was calculated by dividing the number of attributes produced in each category by the total number of attributes used. Statistically speaking, the MANOVA was not reliable, $F(16, 136) = 1.59$, $p = .08$. There were no significant differences in the proportion of *physical traits–lifelong attributes*, *physical traits–disease attributes*, *personal characteristics–lifelong attributes*, *personal characteristics–disease attributes*, *familial attributes*, *vocational attributes*, *educational attributes*, and *talents, hobbies, and interests attributes*. Proportions that exceeded 1% are shown in the Figure A.2. Proportionally speaking, the types of attributes used were similar across all three levels of cognitive impairment.

As with the proportion of attribute use, the proportion of pronoun use was determined by dividing the number of pronouns produced in each of the seven categories by the total number of pronouns used. This MANOVA was reliable, $F(14, 138) = 2.95$, $p < .01$, $\eta^2 = .23$. However, univariate tests revealed no significant differences for the use of *I, myself, my, implicit,* and *plural.* There were significant differences in the proportion of the use of *me, mine,* and *placeholder,* although very small. Proportionally, the types of pronouns used were similar across all three levels of cognitive impairment.

Visual Recognition Data

As hypothesized, there were no differences in visual self-recognition across levels of cognitive impairment. The two test conditions (individual and group) were analyzed separately. Since the differences were small and the responses straightforward, inferential statistics were not employed in these analyses.

Individual test condition. When the participants were shown the photo just taken of them, all of the participants with no cognitive impairments and all participants with mild cognitive impairments self-recognized. Most of those with moderate cognitive impairments (88%) also self-recognized. The three participants who did not self-recognize lived in residential settings. To the question, "Can you tell me who the person in this picture is?," the responses of the three who did not self-recognize were as follows:

- "I have no idea. Maybe it's supposed to be me. If so, I have certainly changed."
- "I don't know. It could be me. It's not me, is it? No."
- "It looks kind of familiar, but I can't place it."

Even among those who successfully self-recognized using the recent photograph of themselves, a number of participants with moderate cognitive impairments volunteered some revealing comments that indicate significant difficulty with recall:

- "I've always hated that picture."
- "I have the same clothes on that I have on today."
- "That was some years ago, though."
- "I don't know when that was taken."
- "When did you take that?"
- "Where did you get that picture?"

Group test condition. All participants in each of the three groups of cognitive impairment correctly self-identified from the group of photos they were shown. After successfully self-recognizing, however, a number of revealing comments were made by participants with mild and moderate cognitive impairments, including:

- "I've always hated that picture."

- "I have the same clothes I have on today."
- "In fact, I think I'm wearing the same shirt."
- "It was taken in this building. It looks like I am wearing the same dress."

Things to Consider When Interpreting the Findings

It should be noted that this study had some limitations that could affect the generalization of the results to all people with AD. The sample was one of convenience and generally represented Caucasian, female, and educated individuals who resided in a metropolitan area. Therefore, the findings cannot be generalized to other populations. The validity and reliability of the visual self-recognition tests and interview guide that were applied have not been established. Finally, the construct of self is a difficult one to measure. Therefore, it is difficult to determine if the measures are truly representative of self.

Future Research

The current study was designed to further examine the persistence of self in individuals with AD. Future research should continue to measure self in individuals with cognitive impairment, both qualitatively and quantitatively, to provide further support. A study that uses an interactive tool or interview guide may create a supportive prosthetic environment for individuals with cognitive impairments to be successful in their communication. A scaffolding approach—adapted from early childhood literature—may also be fruitful in promoting the maintenance of self, and is discussed in Chapter Seven. Most important, research that examines the impact of interactions on the self is very much needed. Investigations of the relation between primary caregiver attitudes and the individual's references to the self may yield some interesting findings regarding the impact of interactions with healthy other adults on the loss or maintenance and display of self. Videotaped interactions between the individual and care provider may also better explore the socially supported self in the moment and its effect on types of attributes. The impact on individuals with dementia could be profound.

References

Addis, D. R., & Tippett, L. J. (2004). Memory of myself: Autobiographical memory and identity in Alzheimer's disease. *Memory, 12*(1), 56–74.

Alzheimer's Association. (2002). *Facts: About Alzheimer's disease* [Brochure]. Chicago: Alzheimer's Disease and Related Disorders Association, Inc.

Alzheimer's Association. (2004). *Statistics* [Brochure]. Chicago: Alzheimer's Disease and Related Disorders Association, Inc.

Alzheimer's Association (2006). Retrieved from www.alz.org.

Alzheimer's Association. (2007). *Alzheimer's disease facts and figures 2007* [Brochure]. Chicago: Alzheimer's Disease and Related Disorders Association, Inc.

American Psychological Association. (2002). Ethical principles of psychologists and code of conduct. *American Psychologist, 47*, 1597–1611.

Baldwin, J. M. (1894). *Mental development in the child and the race.* New Jersey: Macmillan and Co.

Ballenger, J. F. (2006). *Self, senility, and Alzheimer's disease in modern America: A history.* Baltimore: Johns Hopkins University Press.

Baltes, P. B., & Baltes, M. M. (1990). Psychological perspectives on successful aging: A model of selective optimization with compensation. In P. B. Baltes & M. M. Baltes (Eds.), *Successful aging: Perspectives from the behavioral sciences* (pp. 1–34). Cambridge, England: Cambridge University Press.

Bandler, R., & Grinder, J. (1982). *Reframing.* Moab, UT: Real People Press.

Bender, M. (2003). Insight, "inconsistency," and selves. *Explorations in dementia: Theoretical and research studies into the experience of remediable and enduring cognitive losses,* (pp. 238–259). Philadelphia: Jessica Kingsley Publishers.

Benson, M. J., Long, J. K., & Sporakowski, M. J. (1992). Teaching psychopathology and the DSM-III-R from a family systems therapy perspective. *Family Relations, 41*, 135–140.

Biringer, F., & Anderson, J. R. (1992). Self-recognition in Alzheimer's disease: A mirror and video study. *Journal of Gerontology: Psychological Sciences, 47*(6), 385–388.

157

Bjorklund, D. F. (2000). *Children's thinking: Developmental function and individual differences.* Belmont, CA: Wadsworth.

Borkowski, J. G., Benton, A. L., & Spreen, O. (1967). Word fluency and brain damage. *Neuropsychologia, 5,* 135–140.

Brawley, E. C. (1997). *Designing for Alzheimer's disease: Strategies for creating better care environments.* New York: John Wiley & Sons.

Brinthaupt, T. M., & Lipka, R. P. (Eds.). (1992). *The self: Definitional and methodological issues.* Albany, New York: State University of New York Press.

Brooker, D. (2004). What is person-centred care for people with dementia? *Reviews in Clinical Gerontology, 180,* 215–222.

Budson, A. E., & Price, B. H. (2005). Memory dysfunction. *New England Journal of Medicine, 352,* 692–699.

Byrne, B. (1996). *Measuring self-concept across the life span: Issues and instrumentation.* Washington, DC: American Psychological Association.

Calkins, M. P. (2001). *Creating successful dementia care settings.* Baltimore: Health Professions Press.

Calkins, M. P. (2002). The nursing home of the future: Are you ready? *Nursing Homes Long Term Care Management,* June, 43–47.

Calkins, M. P., & Sloane, P. D. (1997). Environment. In *Key Elements of Dementia Care* (67–80). Chicago: Alzheimer's Association.

Callahan, D. (2001). Our need for caring. In L. E. Cluff & R. H. Binstock (Eds.), *The lost art of caring: A challenge to health professionals, families, community, and society,* (pp. 11–24). Baltimore: Johns Hopkins University Press.

Carboni, J. T. (1990). Homelessness among the institutionalized elderly. *Journal of Gerontological Nursing, 16*(7), 32–37.

Cavanuagh, J. C., & Blanchard-Fields, F. (2002). *Adult development and aging.* Belmont, CA: Wadsworth.

Clare, L. (2003). Managing threats to self: Awareness in early stage Alzheimer's disease. *Social Science and Medicine, 57,* 1017–1029.

Cohen, D., & Eisdorfer, C. (1986). *The loss of self.* New York: Norton.

Cohen-Mansfield, J., Golander, H., & Arnheim, G. (2000). Self-identity in older persons suffering from dementia: Preliminary results. *Social Science & Medicine, 51,* 381–394.

Cohen-Mansfield, J., Parpura-Gill, A., & Golander, H. (2006). Utilization of self-identity roles for designing interventions for persons with dementia. *Journal of Gerontology: Psychological Sciences, 61*(4), P202–P212.

Cooley, C. H. (1902). *Human nature and the social order.* New York: Charles Scribner's Sons.

Craik, F. I. M., Moroz, T. M., Moscovitch, M., Stuss, D. T., Winocur, G., Tulving, E., & Kapur, S. (1999). In search of the self: A positron emission tomography study. *Psychological Science, 10*, 26–34.

Csikszentmihalyi, M. (1990). *Flow: The psychology of optimal experience.* New York: Harper & Row.

Damon, W., & Hart, D. (1982). The development of self-understanding from infancy through adolescence. *Child Development, 53*, 848–864.

Downs, M., Clare, L. & Mackenzie, J. (2006). Understanding of dementia: Explanatory models and their implications for the person with dementia and therapeutic effort. In J. C. Hughes, S. J. Louw, & S. R. Sabat (Eds.), *Dementia: Mind, meaning, and the person* (pp. 235–258). New York: Oxford University Press.

Fazio, S., Seman, D., & Stansell, J. (1999). *Rethinking Alzheimer's care.* Baltimore: Health Professions Press.

Fivush, R. (2001). Owning experience: Developing subjective perspective in autobiographical narratives. In C. Moore & K. Lemmon (Eds.), *The self in time: Developmental perspectives* (pp. 35–52). New Jersey: Lawrence Erlbaum Associates, Inc.

Folstein, M. F., Folstein, S. E., & McHugh, P. R. (1975). Mini-Mental State: A practical method for grading the cognitive state of patients for the clinician. *Journal of Psychiatric Research, 12*(3), 189–198.

Fontana, A., & Smith, R. W. (1989). Alzheimer's disease victims: the "unbecoming" of self and the normalization of competence. *Sociological Perspectives, 32*(1), 35–46.

Forstl, H., Besthorn, C., Burns, A., Geiger-Kabisch, C., Levy, R., & Sattel, A. (1994). Delusional misidentification in Alzheimer's disease: A summary of clinical and biological aspects. *Pyschopathology, 27*, 194–199.

Gayle, J. A. (1989). The effect of terminology on public consciousness related to the HIV epidemic. *AIDS Education and Prevention, 1*, 247–250.

Giarrusso, R., Mabry, J. B., Bengston, V. L. (2001). The aging self in social contexts. In R. Binstock (Ed.), *Handbook of aging and the social sciences, fifth edition* (pp. 295–312). San Diego, CA: Academic Press.

Gil, R., Arroyo-Anilo, E. M., Ingrand, P., Gil, M., Neau, J. P., Ornon, C., & Bonnaud, V. (2001). Self-consciousness and Alzheimer's disease. *Acta Neurologica Scandinavica, 104*, 296–300.

Goffman, E. (1959). *The presentation of self in everyday life.* Garden City, NJ: Doubleday.

Goldsmith, M. (1996). *Hearing the voice of people with dementia.* London: Jessica Kingsley Publishers.

Grewal, R. P. (1994). Self-recognition in dementia of the Alzheimer type. *Perceptual and Motor Skills, 79*, 1009–1010.

Harre, R. (1987). The social construction of selves. In K. Yardley & T. Honess (Eds.), *Self and identity: Psychosocial perspectives* (pp. 42–52). Oxford, England: John Wiley & Sons.

Harre, R. (1991). The discursive production of selves. *Theory & Psychology, 1*(1), 51–63.

Harrison, C. (1993). Personhood, dementia, and the integrity of life. *Canadian Journal on Aging, 12*(4), 428–440.

Harter, S. (1988). Developmental processes in the construction of self. In T. D. Yawkey & J. E. Johnson (Eds.), *Integrative processes and socialization: Early to middle childhood* (pp. 45–78). New Jersey: Lawrence Erlbaum Associates, Inc.

Harter, S. (1999). *The construction of the self: A developmental perspective.* New York: Guilford Press.

Herskovits, E. (1995). Struggling over subjectivity: Debates about the self and Alzheimer's disease. *Medical Anthropology Quarterly, 9*(2), 146–164.

Howe, M. L., & Courage, M. L. (1993). On resolving the enigma of infantile amnesia. *Psychological Bulletin, 113*(2), 305–326.

Hubbard, G., Cook, A., Tester, S., & Downs, M. (2002). Beyond words: Older people with dementia using and interpreting nonverbal behaviour. *Journal of Aging Studies, 16*, 155–167.

James, W. (1950). *The Principles of Psychology.* New York: Dover.

Johnson, S. C., Baxter, L. C., Wilder, L. S., Pipe, J. G., Heiserman, J. E., & Prigatano, G. P. (2002). Neural correlates of self-reflection. *Brain, 125*, 1808–1814.

Keenan, J. P., Gallup, G. G., & Falk, D. (2003). *The face in the mirror: The search for the origins of consciousness.* New York: HarperCollins Publishers.

Kitwood, T. (1988). The technical, the personal, and the framing of dementia. *Social Behaviour, 3*, 161–179.

Kitwood, T. (1990). The dialectics of dementia: With particular reference to Alzheimer's disease. *Aging and Society, 10*, 177–196.

Kitwood, T. (1993). *Frames of reference for an understanding of dementia.* Bradford: University of Bradford Research Group.

Kitwood, T. (1997). *Dementia reconsidered: The person comes first.* Buckingham: Open University Press.

Kitwood, T., & Bredin, K. (1992). Towards a theory of dementia care: Personhood and well-being. *Aging and Society, 12*, 269–287.

Kolanowski, A. M., & Whall, A. L. (1996). Life-span perspective of personality in dementia. *IMAGE: Journal of Nursing Scholarship, 28*(4), 315–320.

Lemme, B. H. (1999). *Development in adulthood.* Boston: Allyn and Bacon.

Lewis, M., & Brookes-Gunn, J. (1979). *Social cognition and the acquisition of self.* New York: Plenum Press.

Lewis, M. (1991). Ways of knowing: Objective self-awareness or consciousness. *Developmental Review, 11,* 231–243.

Lipowski, Z. J. (1969). Psychosocial aspects of disease. *Annals of Internal Medicine, 71,* 1191–1206.

Lushin, G. (1990). *The living death: Alzheimer's in America.* United States: The National Foundation for Medical Research.

Lyman, K. A. (1989). Bringing the social back in: A critique of the biomedicalization of dementia. *The Gerontologist, 29,* 597–605.

Lyons, K., Kemper, S., LaBarge, E., Ferraro, F. R., Balota, D., & Storandt, M. (1994). Oral language and Alzheimer's disease: A reduction in syntactic complexity. *Aging and Cognition, 1,* 271–281.

Markova, I. (1987). Knowledge of the self through interaction. In K. Yardley & T. Honess (Eds.), *Self & identity: Psychosocial perspectives* (pp. 65–82). New York: John Wiley & Sons.

McAdams, D. P. (1993). *The stories we live by: Personal myths and the making of the self.* New York: William Morrow.

Mead, G. H. (1925). The genesis of the self and social control. *Child Development, 6,* 251–277.

Mendez, M. F., Martin, R. J., Smyth, K. A., & Whitehouse, P. J. (1992). Disturbances of person identification in Alzheimer's disease: A retrospective study. *Journal of Nervous & Mental Disease, 180,* 94–96.

Molchan, S. E., Martinez, R. A., Lawler, B. A., Grafman, J. H., & Sunderland, T. (1990). Reflections of the self: Atypical misidentification and delusional syndromes in two patients with Alzheimer's disease. *British Journal of Psychiatry, 157,* 605–608.

Morris, R. G. (1996). The neuropsychology of Alzheimer's disease and related dementias. In R. T. Woods (Ed.), *Handbook of the clinical psychology of aging* (pp. 219–242). New York: John Wiley & Sons.

Muller, M. E., & Cox Dzurec, L. (1993). The power of the name. *Advances in Nursing Science, 15*(3), 15–22.

National Institute on Aging. (2003). *Alzheimer's disease: Unraveling the mystery.* Washington, DC: National Institutes of Health.

Nelson, K. (2001). Language and the self: From the "experiencing I" to the "continuing me." In C. Moore & K. Lemmon (Eds.), *The self in time: Developmental perspectives* (pp. 15–34). New Jersey: Lawrence Erlbaum Associates, Inc.

Newman, B. M., & Newman, P. R. (1995). *Development through life: A psychosocial approach.* Pacific Grove, CA: Brookes/Cole Publishing.

P. D. Nussbaum (Ed.). *Handbook of neuropsychology and aging: Critical issues in neuropsychology*. New York: Plenum Press.

Pearce, A., Clare, L., & Pistrang, N. (2002). Managing sense of self. *Dementia, 1*(2), 173–192.

Pelham, B. W., & Hetts, J. J. (1999). Implicit and explicit personal and social identity: Toward a more complete understanding of the social self. In T. R. Tyler, R. M. Kramer, & O. P. John (Eds.), *The psychology of the social self* (pp. 115–143). New Jersey: Lawrence Erlbaum Associates, Inc.

Pesut, D. J. (1991). The art, science, and techniques of reframing in psychiatric mental health nursing. *Issues in Mental Health Nursing, 12*, 9–18.

Petersen, R. (2002). *Mayo Clinic on Alzheimer's disease*. New York: Kensington Publishing.

Pioneer Network. (2006). Retrieved from www.pioneernetwork.net.

Povinelli, D. J. (1995). The unduplicated self. In Rochat, P. (Ed.) *The self in infancy: Theory and research* (pp. 161–192). Amsterdam: Elsevier Science B.V.

Povinelli, D. J. (2001). The self: Elevated in consciousness and extended in time. In C. Moore & K. Lemmon (Eds.), *The self in time: Developmental perspectives* (pp. 75–96). New Jersey: Lawrence Erlbaum Associates, Inc.

Robertson, A. (1991). The politics of Alzheimer's disease: A case study in apocalyptic demography. In M. Minkler & C. L. Estes (Eds.), *Critical perspectives on Aging: The political and moral economy of growing old* (pp. 135–150). New York: Baywood Publishing Company.

Ross, A. O. (1992). *The sense of self: Research and theory*. New York: Springer Publishing.

Ryden, M. B. (1998). A theory of caring and dementia. *American Journal of Alzheimer's Disease*, July/August, 203–207.

Sabat, S. R. (2002). Surviving manifestations of selfhood in Alzheimer's disease. *Dementia, 1*(1), 25–36.

Sabat, S. (2006). Mind, meaning, and personhood in dementia: The effects of positioning. In J. C. Hughes, S. J. Louw, & S. R. Sabat (Eds.), *Dementia: Mind, meaning, and the person* (287–302). New York: Oxford University Press.

Sabat, S. R., & Collins, M. (1999). Intact social, cognitive ability, and selfhood: A case study of Alzheimer's disease. *American Journal of Alzheimer's Disease*, January/February, 11–19.

Sabat, S. R., & Harre, R. (1992). The construction and deconstruction of self in Alzheimer's disease. *Aging and Society, 12*, 443–461.

Salmon, D. P., & Bondi, M. W. (1997). The neuropsychology of Alzheimer's disease. In P. D. Nussbaum (Ed.), *Handbook of neuropsychology and aging: Critical issues in neuropsychology* (pp. 141–158). New York: Plenum Press.

Schaie, K. W., & Willis, S. L. (1996). *Adult development and aging.* New York: Harper-Collins.

Seman, D. (2002). Meaningful communication throughout the journey. In P. B. Harris (Ed.), *The person with Alzheimer's disease: Pathways to understanding the experience* (pp. 134–149). Baltimore: Johns Hopkins University Press.

Shaffer, D. R. (2002). *Developmental Psychology.* Belmont, CA: Wadsworth.

Shenk, D. (2001). *The forgetting: Alzheimer's: Portrait of an epidemic.* New York: Doubleday.

Shenk, D., Davis, B., Peacock, J. R., & Moore, L. (2002). Narratives and self-identity in later life: Two rural American older women. *Journal of Aging Studies, 16,* 401–413.

Small, J. A., Geldart, K., Gutman, G., & Clarke Scott, M. A. (1998). The discourse of self in dementia. *Aging and Society, 18,* 291–316.

St. George-Hyslop, P. H. (2000). Piecing together Alzheimer's. *Scientific American, 283*(6), 76–83.

Stetsenko, A., & Arievitch, I. (1997). Constructing and deconstructing the self: Comparing Post-Vgotskian and discourse-based versions of social constructivism. *Mind, Culture, and Activity, 4*(3), 159–172.

Surr, C. A. (2006). Preservation of self in people with dementia living in residential care: A socio-biographical approach. *Social Science & Medicine, 62,* 1720–1730.

Swanson-Kauffman, K. M. (1986). Caring in the instance of unexpected early pregnancy loss. *Topics in Clinical Nursing, 8*(2), 37–46.

Taft, L., Delaney, K., Seman, D., & Stansell, J. (1993). Dementia care: Creating a therapeutic milieu. *Journal of Gerontological Nursing,* October, 30–39.

Taft, L. B., Fazio, S., Seman D., & Stansell, J. (1997). A psychosocial model of dementia care: Theoretical and empirical support. *Archives of Psychiatric Nursing, 11*(1), 13–20.

Tappen, R., Williams, C., Fishman, S., & Touhy, T. (1999). Persistence of self in advanced Alzheimer's disease. *Journal of Nursing Scholarship, 31*(2), 121–125.

TLC in LTC of Illinois. (2006). Retrieved from www.tlcinltc.org.

Turner, J. C., & Onorato, R. S. (1999). Social identity, personality, and the self-concept: A self-categorization perspective. In T. R. Tyler, R. M. Kramer, O. P. John (Eds.), *The psychology of the social self* (pp. 11–46). New Jersey: Lawrence Erlbaum Associates, Inc.

Watson, J. (1988). *Nursing: Human science and human care.* New York: National League for Nursing.

Whitbourne, S. K. (1987). Personality development in adulthood and old age: Relationships among identity style, health, and well-being. In K. W. Schaie (Ed.), *Annual review of gerontology and geriatrics,* Vol. 7, pp. 186–216. New York: Springer.

Zingmark, K., Norberg, A., & Sandman, P. (1993). Experiences of at-homeness and homesickness in patients with Alzheimer's disease. *The American Journal of Alzheimer's Care and Related Disorders and Research*, May/June, 10–16.

Zingmark, K., Norberg, A., & Sandman, P. (1995). The experiences of being at home throughout the life span: Investigation of persons aged from 2 to 102. *International Journal of Aging and Human Development*, *41*(1), 47–62.

RECOMMENDED READINGS

Before training, his mind was like a stag with great antlers trying to make its way through a thick forest; the animal got snagged on branches time after time. But after many years of practice, his mind was more like a monkey in a jungle, swinging freely from vine to vine.

Tibetan Lama

As you may have noticed from my writing, my professional and personal influences vary greatly and include both conventional and unconventional resources. I have found that in order to broaden my thinking about and approaches to care, I also need to broaden my influences. I present the resources that follow as examples of that broadening, and to serve as springboards for you as you, too, expand your influences and thinking.

Alzheimer's Disease and Care

Ballenger, J. F. (2006). *Self, senility, and Alzheimer's disease in modern America: A history.* Baltimore: Johns Hopkins University Press.

Bell, V. & Troxel, D. (1997). *The best friends approach to Alzheimer's care.* Baltimore: Health Professions Press.

Calkins, M. P. (2001). *Creating successful dementia care settings.* Baltimore: Health Professions Press.

Davidson, A. (1997). *Alzheimer's, a love story: One year in my husband's journey.* Secaucus, NJ: Carol Publishing.

Fazio, S., Seman, D., & Stansell, J. (1999). *Rethinking Alzheimer's care.* Baltimore: Health Professions Press.

Goldsmith, M. (1996). *Hearing the voice of people with dementia.* London: Jessica Kingsley Publishers.

Harding, N., & Palfrey, C. (1997). *The social construction of dementia: Confused professionals.* Bristol, PA: Jessica Kingsley Publishers.

Harris, P. B. (Ed.) (2002). *The person with Alzheimer's disease: Pathways to understanding the experience.* Pages 134–149. Baltimore: Johns Hopkins University Press.

Hughes, J. C., Louw, S. J., & Sabat, S. R. (Eds.) (2006). *Dementia: Mind, meaning, and the person.* Pages 287–302. New York: Oxford University Press.

Kitwood, T. (1997). *Dementia reconsidered: The person comes first.* Buckingham, England: Open University Press.

Mitchell, M. (2002). *Dancing on quicksand: A gift of friendship on the age of Alzheimer's.* Boulder, CO: Johnson Books.

Rader, J. (1995). *Individualized dementia care: Creative, compassionate approaches.* New York: Springer Publishing.

Caring

Brandon, D. (1990). *Zen in the art of helping.* New York: Arkana.

Cluff, L. E., & Binstock, R. H. (2001). *The lost art of caring: A challenge to health professionals, families, community, and society.* Pages 11–24. Baltimore: Johns Hopkins University Press.

Frankl, V. E. (1986). *The doctor and the soul.* New York: Vintage Books.

Lustbader, W. (1991). *Counting on kindness: The dilemmas of dependency.* New York: The Free Press.

Mayeroff, M. (1971). *On caring.* New York: Harper Perennial.

Social Sciences

Csikszentmihalyi, M. (1990). *Flow: The psychology of optimal experience.* New York: Harper & Row.

Goffman, E. (1959). *The presentation of self in everyday life.* Garden City, NJ: Doubleday.

Goffman, E. (1963). *Stigma.* Englewood Cliffs, NJ: Prentice Hall.

Soul, Sacredness, Mindfulness, and Zen Practices

Carlson, R., & Shield, B. (Eds.) (1995). *Handbook for the soul.* Boston: Little, Brown and Company.

Carse, J. P. (1994). *Breakfast at the victory: The mysticism of ordinary experience.* New York: Harper San Francisco.

Das, S. (1997). *Awaking the Buddha within.* New York: Broadway Books.

Frankl, V. E. (1959). *Man's search for meaning.* New York: Washington Square Press.

Gunaratana, V. H. (1994). *Mindfulness in plain English.* Boston: Wisdom Publications.

Hayward, J. (1995). *Sacred world.* New York: Bantam Books.

Jackson, P., & Delehanty, H. (1995). *Sacred hoops: Spiritual lessons of a hardwood warrior.* New York: Hyperion.

Kabat-Zinn, J. (1994). *Wherever you go, there you are: Mindfulness meditation in everyday life.* New York: Hyperion.

Kushner, L. (1996). *Invisible lines of connection: Sacred stories of the ordinary.* Woodstock, VT: Jewish Lights Publishing.

Moore, T. (1992). *Care of the soul: A guide for cultivating depth and sacredness in everyday life.* New York: HarperCollins.

Moore, T. (1996). *The education of the heart.* New York: HarperCollins.

Reps, P., & Senzaki, N. (1998). *Zen flesh, Zen bones.* Boston: Tuttle Publishing.

Suzuki, S. (1970). *Zen mind, beginner's mind.* New York: Weatherhill.

Toole, E. (1999). *The power of now: A guide to spiritual enlightenment.* Novato, CA: New World Library.

INDEX

Note: AD stands for Alzheimer's disease throughout the index

Abandonment, fear of, 87
Abstract thinking, problems with, 44
Activities, 92–94, 128–129
    clustering to organize care and, 91–92
    defined, 92
    domains of, 92, 93, 96
    flexible structure of, 93
    grading of, 93–94
    providing, within an environment, 92–94
Activity-Based Alzheimer Care (ABAC) program, 92–94
Adaptation, 39–40
Addis, D. R., 37
Adult day centers, 48
Alzheimer's Association, 50
    Dementia Care Conference of 2006, 124
Alzheimer's disease (AD). *See also* Dementia
    care environments, 48–49
    causes of, 45
    diagnosis of, 45–46
    emerging thinking in AD care, 50
    evidence of self in, *see* Evidence of self in AD
    models of care, *see* Person-centered care; Traditional medical model
    myths about, examining, 52
    overview of, 43–56, 139–140
    rate of progression, 43, 46
    stages and progression of, 46–47, 53–56
    statistics, 43
    support, sources for, 50
    symptoms of, 43, 44–45
    time of onset until death, 43
    treatments for, 47–48
Alzheimer's Family Care Center, xi

Anderson, J. R., 59, 65
Anxiety, 48
Apprentice in thinking, 118
Approaches to care and intervention, 88–91
    behavioral, 90
    cognitive, 90–91
    environmental, 90
    functional, 89–90
    medical, 90
    psychological, 89
    social, 89
Aromatherapy, 86
Assisted living, 48–49
Attachment, 7
Autobiographical memory, 37
Autonomy, 20–21

Baldwin, J. M., 36
Ballenger, J. F., 109
Baltes, M. M., 40
Baltes, P. B., 40
Basting, Anne, 57, 124
Bathrooms, 79
Behavioral approaches to care and interventions, 90
Being in the moment, 107, 120–121
    caring moments, 122–123
    Zen practices for, 130
Bender, M., 61
Bengston, V. L., 35
Biography, sharing of person's, *see* Learning about the person
Biography boards, 76
Biringer, F., 59, 65
Blanchard-Fields, F., 38–39
Body language (nonverbal behavior), 61, 106. *See also* Language
Brawley, Elizabeth, 8, 78, 79, 80

Bredin, K., 5, 6, 7, 102–103
Brooker, D., 8
Brooks-Gunn, J., 35

Calkins, Margaret, 75, 78, 95
Callahan, D., 16
Carboni, J. T., 80
Caregivers. *See also* Person-centered care
    approaches to care and intervention, *see*
        Approaches to care and intervention
    care environments, *see* Physical environ-
        ment; Social and cultural
        environments
    implementing change, *see* Implementing
        change
    principles for providing person-centered
        care, *see* Principles for providing
        person-centered care, Kitwood's
    relationships and interactions with, *see*
        Relationships and interactions that
        support the self
    sharing key points with other staff, 136–
        148
    taking action toward change, 133–136
Caring
    communication and, *see* Communication
    deeper level involvement in, 17
    focus on connecting, not correcting,
        17–18
    listening when, *see* Listening
    for the person, not the disease, 16–17
    processes involved in, 15–16
Caring community, 19–20
Cavanaugh, J. C., 38–39
Celebration, 86
Cerebral cortex, 45
Change, implementing, *see* Implementing
    change
Chavin, Melanie, 92
Choices, *see* Control issues
Cholinesterase inhibitors, 47
Clare, L., 116
Clifton Assessment Procedures for the Elderly,
    61
Clustering to organize care and activities,
    91–92
Cognitive approaches to care and interventions,
    90–91
Cognitive function
    AD and impairment of, 43
    hyper-cognitive culture, 102
    judging a person by, ix–x, 58, 102
Cohen-Mansfield, J., 64, 125
Collaboration with person with dementia, 85

Collins, M., 25, 60, 62, 124
Comfort, 7
Communication. *See also* Language
    building a caring relationship through,
        104–106, 112
    listening, *see* Listening
    meeting the pace of person being cared for,
        105–106
    nonverbal, 61, 106
    soulful connections, 106–110
Control issues, 20
    disempowerment, 101
    empowerment, 119
    physical environment and personal con-
        trol, 77, 79, 81
    validation in a therapeutic milieu, 83
Cooley, C. H., 36
Creating Successful Dementia Care Settings
    (Calkins), 78
Creutzfeldt-Jakob disease, 44
Csikszentmihalyi, M., 120
Cultural environment, *see* Social and cultural
    environments
Culture change movement, 7–11. *See also*
    Person-centered care

Dementia
    AD as form of, *see* Alzheimer's disease
        (AD)
    causes, besides AD, 44
    global states of, 6
    indicators of well-being, 6
    with Lewy bodies, 44
    medical approach to, *see* Traditional med-
        ical model
    mixed, 44
    vascular, 44
Dementia care mapping, 7
Dependency, 102
Depersonalization, 14, 100–101
    with words and labels, 12–13, 58
Design Innovations for Aging and Alzheimer's
    (Brawley), 8
Design of physical environment for dementia
    care, *see* Physical environment
Diamond, Marian, 5
Dignity, 20
Disorientation, 44
Disruptive behaviors, design of physical envi-
    ronment to minimize, 78
Domains of self, 31, 111
Downs, M., 8
Drug treatments for AD and dementia, 47, 48,
    90

Eden alternative, 9
Emotions, 107–108
Empowerment, 119
Environments, care, *see* Physical environment; Social and cultural environments
Everyday care, supporting the self in, 115–132, 147–148
  being in the moment, 120–121
  caring moments, 122–123
  evolving self, supporting the, 117, 129
  experiencing flow, 119–120
  illustration of care that maintains self, 125–129
  maintaining a sense of self, 115–116, 131–132
  prosthetic or supportive environment, creating a, 117–119
  self-identity and interventions, 125
Evidence of self in AD, 57–71, 141–142
  narrative techniques, 37, 60–62, 63–65
  new research on, 62–70
  qualitative analyses, 66–70
  typical portrayals of AD, 58–59
  visual self-recognition techniques, 37, 59, 65–66
Evolving self, 38–39, 115–116, 117, 123–124, 129

Facilitation of accomplishments of person with dementia, 88
Fagan, Rose Marie, ix
Family
  person-centered care, *see* Person-centered care
  relationships and interactions with, *see* Relationships and interactions that support the self
Fazio, Sam, ix, x, 15, 20, 115
  Activity-Based Alzheimer Care (ABAC) program, 92–94
  development of approach toward dementia care, xi–xii
Fivush, R., 35
Flexible structure, 93
Flow, 119–120
Food and Drug Administration, U.S. (FDA), 47
Free radicals, 47
Friends
  person-centered care, *see* Person-centered care
  relationships and interactions with, *see* Relationships and interactions that support the self
Froggatt, 64

Frontotemporal dementia, 44
Functional magnetic resonance imaging (fMRI), 66
Functional approaches to care and interventions, 89–90

Gardens, 79
Giarusso, R., 35
Gil, R., 37, 59
Global Deterioration Scale, 59
Glutamate, 47
Goffman, E., 36
Golas, Thaddeus, 133
Goldsmith, M., 104, 105–106, 119, 124
Green House Project, 9
Grewal, R. P., 59
Group-type homes, 48–49
Gubrium, Jaber, 106
Guided participation, 118
Gunderson, John, 82

Hallucinations, 48
Harre, R., 37, 60, 61, 62, 99
Harrison, C., 58
Harter, S., 36–37
Herbal remedies, 48
Herskovits, E., 58, 61
Hetts, J. J., 36
Hippocampus, 45, 66
Holding of person with dementia, 87–88
Holding onto Home (Cohen and Weisman), 78, 79
Holistic care, 49, 50
Home, identity and feeling of, 80–81
Home care, 48
Humor, 107
Hyper-cognitive culture, 102

I-assessment, 26
Ideal or possible self, 41
Identity, 7, 124
  components of, 34
  designing individualized interventions, 125
  design of physical environment to maintain, 77, 78, 79–80
  development through adulthood, 38–39, 115–116, 117, 123–124
  home and, feeling of, 80–81
  personal versus social, 99–100
Illness model, *see* Traditional medical model
Implementing change, 133–136
  build a support system, 135–36
  develop an action plan, 134–135
  evaluate and revise, 136

Implementing change (*continued*)
  meet with leadership, 134
  review materials and resources, 133–134
  reward change and celebrate success, 135
  share the learning, 135
Inclusion, 7, 119
Independence, design of physical environment
    to support, 78
Infantilism, 101
Initiative, loss of, 45
Interdependence, 102
Internet resources, 50
Intimidation of person with dementia, 101
Involvement in a therapeutic milieu, 83
Invulnerable self, 40

James, William, 34–35, 38
Johnson, S. C., 66
Judgment, poor or decreased, 44
Just Right Challenge, 118

Kaufman, Sharon, 39
Keenan, J. P., 39
Key Elements of Dementia Care (Calkins and
    Sloane), 75
Kitwood, Tom, ix, 5, 7, 8, 20, 36, 50, 58, 99,
    102–103
  on communication, 105
  on depersonalizing process, 100–101
  environment and brain function, 5
  Personhood Affirmation Components, 7,
    28
  principles of person-centered care, 83–89,
    97
  rejection of standard medical approach to
    dementia, 5–6
  timalation, coining of term, 86
Kolanowski, A. M., 62

Labeling, 12–13, 101
Language. *See also* Communication; Nonverbal
    behavior
  to describe AD, 58
  impact of words, 12–15, 29, 58
  impairment, as symptom of AD, 43, 44
  person-centered, 11–15
  pronoun use, 61, 64, 124
  to represent self, 37–38, 60–62, 63–65
Learned helplessness, 119
Learning about the person, 21–26, 30–32, 102,
    123–124, 126–127
Lemme, B. H., 33, 34, 39–40
Lewis, M., 35

Life story and maintenance of self, 123–124,
    129
Life-story book, 26
Listening
  building a caring relationship through,
    104, 105, 112
  for meaning, 18–19
Living in the moment, 107, 120–121
  caring moments, 122–123
  Zen practices for, 130
Locke, John, 34
Lubinski, Rosemary, 119
Lyman, Karen, 14, 58

Mabry, J. V., 35
McAdams, Dan, 38–39, 123
MacRae, Hazel, 39
Maintaining a sense of self in everyday care,
    115–116, 131–132
Malignant social positioning, 100–102
Malignant social psychology, 6–7, 100
Markova, I., 39
Massage, 86
Mather LifeWays Institute of Aging, 118
Mead, G. H., 36
Medical (pharmacological) approaches to care
    and interventions, 47, 48, 90
Medicalization of deviance, 58
Medical model of dementia, *see* Traditional
    medical model
Memantine, 47
Memory loss, 43, 44
  autobiographical memory, 37
  caregiver's role in filling in for, 103, 118–
    119
  episodic memory, 66
Mirror-recognition techniques, 37, 59, 65
Misplacing things, 44
Mixed dementia, 44
Moment, being in the, 107, 120–121
  caring moments, 122–123
  Zen practices for, 130
Mood changes, 45

Narrative
  life story and maintenance of self, 123–124
  techniques to study self in AD, 37, 60–62
Needs, basic human, 21
Negative social positioning, 100–102
Negotiation with person with dementia, 85
Nelson, K., 35
Newman, B. M, 34
Newman, P. R., 34

N-methyl-D-aspartate (NMDA) receptor agonists, 47
Noise in the physical environment, 76
Nonverbal behavior, 61, 106. *See also* Language
Nursing home care, 49
    goals for future, 78
Nursing home model, ix, 8

Objectification, 14, 101
Occupation, 7
Onorato, R. S., 36
Osler, Dr. William, 17

Parkinson's disease, 44
Pearce, A., 115
Pelham, B. W., 36
Personality changes, dramatic, 45
Person-centered care, 49
    caring and, 15–20
    core values in providing, 20–21
    culture change movement and, 7–11
    everyday applications, *see* Everyday care, supporting the self in
    getting to know the person, 21–26, 30–32, 102, 123–24, 126–127
    implementing change, *see* Implementing change
    Kitwood's principles for providing, 83–89, 97
    language, person-centered, 11–15
    personhood and the impetus of, 5–7
    physical environment and, *see* Physical environment
    relationships and interactions that support the self, *see* Relationships and interactions that support the self
    the self as the core of, 5–33
    social and cultural environments, *see* Social and cultural environments
    summary, 26–27, 137–138
Personhood Affirmation Components, Kitwood's, 7, 28
Person-work, 103
Photographs, self-recognition in, 62, 65, 66
Physical environment, 75–81, 90, 95, 127–128
    adapting to the disease continuum, 78–79
    awareness and orientation, maximizing, 76, 79
    brain function and, 5
    disruptive behaviors, minimizing, 78
    feeling of home and identity, 80–81
    functional abilities, supporting, 76, 79

    functional independence, supporting, 78
    personal control, providing opportunities for, 77, 79, 81
    privacy, 76, 79, 81
    public spaces, 79
    safety and security of, 76, 79, 81
    self-identity, maintaining, 77, 78
    social contact, facilitating, 77, 79
    stimulation and, 76–77, 79
    summary, 94, 143–144
    therapeutic milieu, elements of a, 82–83
    types of care environments, 48–49
Piaget, Jean, 39
Pioneer Network, ix, 10
    traditional medical model compared with Pioneer Model, 11
    values of, 10
Planetree Model, 9
Play, 85–86
Post, Stephen, ix–x, 102
Povinelli, D. J., 35, 37
Principles for providing person-centered care, Kitwood's, 83–89, 97
    celebration, 86
    collaboration, 85
    facilitation, 88
    holding, 87–88
    negotiation, 85
    play, 85–86
    recognition, 84–85
    relaxation, 86–87
    timalation, 86
    validation, 87
Principles of Psychology (James), 34–35
Privacy, physical environment and, 76, 79, 81
Pronoun use, 61, 64, 124
Prosthetic or supportive environment, creating a, 117–119
Psychological approaches to care and interventions, 89

Recognition of person with dementia, 84–85
Reframing, 14
Regenerative community model, 9
Reisberg, Dr. Barry, 46
Relationships and interactions that support the self, 99–112
    developmental phases of relationships, 103–104
    listening and communication, 104–106, 112
    negative social positioning, 100–102
    the relationship-based approach, 103–104

role of others in person-centered care, 102–103
six domains of self, 111
social construction of the self, 99–102
soulful connections, 106–110
summary, 110, 145–146
Relaxation, 86–87
Research method and results, 149–155
coding, 151
considerations when interpreting findings, 155
future research, 155
language data results, 151–153
materials used, 149–150
participants, 149
procedures, 151
qualitative analyses, 66–70
visual recognition data results, 154–155
Resident-directed care, 9
Residential environment, see Physical environment
Respect, 20
Respite camps, 48
Restraint-free/individualized care, 9
Rethinking Alzheimer's Care (Fazio, Seman, and Stansell), xi, 15, 20, 22, 80, 82, 84
Robertson, A., 58
Rogers, Carl, 8
Rogoff, Barbara, 118
Rooms in care environments, 127–128
décor, 79
entry design, 76
images and objects meaningful to the resident, 77, 79
Ryff, Carol, 41

Sabat, Steven, ix, 25, 47, 50, 60, 61, 62, 99, 124
negative social positioning and, 100–101
Safety
environmental design and, 76, 79, 81
in a therapeutic milieu, 82
Scaffolding, 118
Schaie, K. W., 41
Security, environmental design and, 76, 81
Selective optimization with compensation (SOC), 40
Self
adaptation and, in older adults, 39–40
definitions of, 33, 34
domains of, 31, 111
evidence of, in AD, see Evidence of self in AD
ideal or possible, 41
invulnerable, 40

maintaining a sense of, 115–116
measurements of, 37–38
multidimensional nature of, 33, 35, 42
overview of, 33–42, 139
physical environments that recognize the, see Physical environment
relationships and interactions that support the, see Relationships and interactions that support the self
self-concept and evolving self, 38–39, 115–116, 117, 123–124, 129
social and cultural environments that recognize the, see Social and cultural environments
social construction of the, 36–37, 99–102
theories of early development and, 34–35
Self-awareness, 34, 35
Self-consciousness, 34
Self-identity, see Identity
Self-knowledge, 34, 37
Seman, Dorothy, 15, 20, 104–105
Shenk, David, 8, 64, 100
Shields, Steve, ix
Skills, retained, 21
Sloane, P. D., 75, 95
Small, J. A., 61, 64
Social and cultural environments, 75, 128. See also Relationships and interactions that support the self
activities, see Activities
approaches to care and intervention, see Approaches to care and intervention
clustering to organize care and activities, 91–92
facilitation of social contact, physical space and, 77
feeling of home and, 80–81
principles of person-centered care, Kitwood's, 83–89, 97
prosthetic or supportive environment, creating a, 117–119
summary, 94, 143–144
therapeutic milieu, elements of a, 82–83
Social construction of the self, 36–37, 60, 99–102
Soulful connections, 106–110
Stansell, Jane, 15, 20, 82
Stigmatization, 101
Stimulation
physical environment and, 76–77, 79
timalation, 86
Stories
life story and maintenance of the self, 123–124

life-story book, 26
StoryCorps Memory Loss Initiative, 124
Structure in a therapeutic milieu, 82
Supportive encouragement, 118
Surr, C. A., 102, 123, 124
Swanson-Kaufman, Kristen, 15–16
Symbolic interactionism, 36

Taft, Lois, 82, 88, 90, 97
Tappen, R., 61
Tennessee Self Concept Scale, 37
Therapeutic milieu, elements of a, 82–83
    involvement, 83
    safety, 82
    structure, 82
    support, 82–83
    validation, 83
Timalation, 86
TimeSlips project, 124
Tippett, L. J., 37
Traditional medical model, 5–6, 13–14, 49, 58, 59
    physical needs, focus on, ix, 6
    Pioneer Model compared with, 11

Turner, J. C., 36
Twenty Statements Test, 37

Validation, 87
    invalidation, 101
    in a therapeutic milieu, 83
Vascular dementia, 44
Ventrezio, Maria Rose, 125–129
Video self-recognition techniques, 59
Visual self-recognition techniques, 37, 59, 62, 65–66
Vitamin E supplements, 47
Vygotsky, Lev, 118

Wellspring Model, 9
Whall, A. L., 62
Whitbourne, S. K., 39
Willis, S. L., 41

Zgola, Jitka, 93
Zone of proximal development, 118